Cognitive Behavioral Therapy

Made Simple

Cognitive Behavioral Therapy

Made Simple

10 STRATEGIES

for Managing Anxiety, Depression, Anger, Panic, and Worry

ALTHEA
PRESS

QUICK-START GUIDE

Is this book for you? Read the statements below and check the box if that statement often describes how you feel.

- ❏ I dread the next anxiety attack.
- ❏ I have trouble sleeping.
- ❏ I worry needlessly about many things.
- ❏ I feel tense and anxious and I have a hard time relaxing.
- ❏ Certain objects or situations terrify me.
- ❏ I avoid things I need to do because they make me anxious.
- ❏ I feel extremely nervous in some social situations or avoid them if I can.
- ❏ My angry responses seem overblown for the situation.
- ❏ I don't understand why I feel so angry.
- ❏ My anger has caused problems in my relationships.
- ❏ I can't get interested in things I used to enjoy.
- ❏ I feel like I have nothing to look forward to.
- ❏ I struggle to concentrate and make decisions.
- ❏ I don't like myself.
- ❏ It's hard to find the energy and motivation I need.

If you checked several of the boxes, you can benefit from this book. Read on to learn about CBT and how you can take part of the therapeutic process into your own hands.

For Marcia, with love and gratitude for sharing this life with me.

Contents

Foreword viii

Introduction xii

CHAPTER ONE Your CBT Starter Guide 2

CHAPTER TWO Goal Setting 18

CHAPTER THREE Activate Behavior 32

CHAPTER FOUR Identify and Break Negative Thought Patterns 52

CHAPTER FIVE Identify and Change Your Core Beliefs 70

CHAPTER SIX Maintain Mindfulness 86

CHAPTER SEVEN Stay on Task: Push Through Procrastination 104

CHAPTER EIGHT Work Through Worry, Fear, and Anxiety 120

CHAPTER NINE Keep Calm: Manage Excessive Anger 142

CHAPTER TEN Be Kind to Yourself 158

CONCLUSION Keeping It Going 182

Resources 188

References 196

Index 211

Foreword

Cognitive behavioral therapy (CBT), a powerful psychological treatment, is rooted in a coherent, comprehensive theory of emotions as well as the behaviors connected to those emotions. The theory can guide the discovery of the sources of each individual person's emotional difficulties. Just as important are the tools of CBT, derived from the theory that practitioners have developed over the past 40 years. This great variety of techniques allows therapists to tailor their interventions to the specific needs and preferences of each patient. So how can the power of CBT, which would seem to require a skilled therapist to help patients identify their unique patterns and to select and adapt the right tools, be conveyed in book form? Enter Dr. Seth Gillihan, who in clear and plain yet elegant language is able to connect with any reader who wants to understand and address his or her own barriers to good mental health.

The soothing and confident voice behind this book is one I know very well. In 2005, Seth became the 50th PhD student at the University of Pennsylvania (Penn) whom I taught and supervised in a yearlong practical course in CBT. Over the past 35 years I have been privileged to teach the principles and practice of CBT to some of the most impressive and motivated young professionals one could hope to meet. Their level of talent and knowledge, along with their commitment to learn, continues to amaze me. But Seth left a lasting impression on me for his wisdom and ability to connect to individuals from all backgrounds and walks of life. He possesses an unparalleled ability to convey the best of what I learned from my own mentors, Drs. Steven Hollon and Aaron T. Beck, and he has added extremely useful insights of his own.

I first encountered Seth's gift as a helping professional while watching video recordings of his therapy sessions, reading his case notes, and hearing his crystal-clear descriptions of the successes—and hiccups—he and his clients experienced as they worked together. I now see the same Seth Gillihan, with vastly more experience, who has "warmed up" to the current project by authoring *Retrain Your Brain: Cognitive Behavioral Therapy in 7 Weeks*, a fine workbook, and also coauthoring a practical and sensitive guide for individuals and the families of those who suffer from obsessive-compulsive disorder.

His newest book is a delightful read, which is no small accomplishment given the seriousness of the subject matter and his honest, realistic treatment of the problems he addresses. The book manages to cover a lot of ground, in detail, and yet remain "simple," as its title suggests. It draws even further upon Seth's strengths, including an unmatched ability to organize and structure material, which makes it easy to grasp and retain the many nuggets found within its pages. Unique to this book is the rhythm that Seth establishes at the outset and carries though each chapter, spelling out how to address unhelpful thinking, how to use behaviors to alter problematic patterns, and finally, how to attend to, and be mindful of, the important things in our lives. I was so impressed by this rhythm that I now include it in my own teaching: Think, Act, and Be. What could be simpler? And yet the ideas these words reflect are rich and powerful enough to produce seismic positive shifts in the lives of clients in therapy. They can do the same for readers of this book.

Even if a reader does not have difficulties in all the areas covered in the book (sadness, worry, fear, anger, procrastination, self-criticism), I highly recommend the sections on three topics in particular: procrastination, anger, and "safety behaviors." The insights Seth provides about these often-puzzling yet all-too-common patterns are really interesting! And if nothing else, his characterizations of these patterns can help the reader understand a bit better how they trip up friends, colleagues, or family members.

Most of us procrastinate, yet we do not have insight into the sources of or the processes behind procrastination. Anger, inappropriate or excessive versions of which are all too common, can be understood. This is half the battle in getting anger under our control or in helping a partner who is in its grip. Finally, safety behaviors prevent those with unrealistic fears or compulsive behaviors from breaking free and enjoying what life has to offer. Reading Seth's analysis of these patterns is revelatory and engaging. This is a great example, well explained, of the progress made by psychologists in our understanding of "what makes people tick."

Some readers will turn to this book to brush up on the principles and practices of CBT they had encountered in personal therapy or in another form. Others will learn about CBT for the first time and find all they need to free themselves from unnecessary and unproductive emotional distress and be set on a path to better living. This book can also serve as a much-needed first step for those with more severe problems who have considered taking antidepressant or antianxiety medications or who have tried them and not found them to be helpful, as well as for those who haven't been able to find a therapist they are ready to work with. Many such people will find everything they need within these pages. There will also be others who will begin to learn about the sources and remedies for emotional difficulties that have held them back and kept them from enjoying life, and this will motivate them to seek appropriate professional guidance or help. They can carry what they have learned from Seth and from engaging in the exercises in this book into individual or group therapy if that is the right next step.

Let me sum up by reflecting on how lucky I was to have had the opportunity to contribute to Seth's growth as a psychologist. It is now your luck that you have encountered this truly helpful and (I'll say it again) really interesting guide to common emotional problems and effective ways to overcome them. I urge you to take advantage of this bit of luck and set yourself on a path to better living.

Robert J. DeRubeis, PhD.
Samuel H. Preston Term Professor in the
Social Sciences and Professor of Psychology
School of Arts and Sciences
University of Pennsylvania

Introduction

At some point, all of us will find ourselves in the tight grip of overwhelming emotions. It might be a feeling of anxious dread, depression that drains the color from life, panic that strikes at the most inopportune times, frequent and excessive anger, or other experiences that grip our minds and hearts. When we're knocked off balance emotionally, we need tried and tested ways to regain our footing and find relief as quickly as possible.

Early in my clinical training, I learned that some types of treatment have a lot more evidence to back them up, especially cognitive behavioral therapy (CBT). My first therapy supervisor encouraged me to pursue specialized training in CBT, which led me to the University of Pennsylvania, a school with a rich history in cognitive and behavioral treatments. As I focused on treatment for depression during my doctoral training, I saw how depression bends our thinking in harmful directions, and how CBT can retrain our thoughts to serve us better. I also learned that building more rewarding activities into our lives could have powerful anti-depressant effects.

When I finished my PhD, I was excited to take a faculty position at the university's Center for the Treatment and Study of Anxiety, which had developed many of the best treatments for anxiety. During my four years there, I received intensive experience in treating debilitating anxiety, obsessive-compulsive disorder, and trauma. I saw hundreds of lives changed by treatment programs that helped people face their fears head-on. While I was there I learned that focusing our attention on the present with openness and curiosity is a powerful way to break the grip of anxiety and depression. This mindfulness-based approach has gained sufficient research support to warrant its status as the "third wave" of CBT, alongside cognitive and behavioral techniques.

Over the past two decades as a student, researcher, therapist, and supervisor, two things have stood out to me about effective treatments. Number one, they're simple: *Do enjoyable activities. Think helpful thoughts. Face your fears. Be present. Take care of yourself.* None of these approaches is shocking or complicated. I've strived to capture that simplicity in the chapters ahead. When we're struggling, we typically don't have the time, desire, or energy to wade through page after page of research findings or study a treatise on the esoteric nuances in the field. We need straight-forward options we can use right away.

Number two, they're not easy. I've learned that despite the simplicity of these effective treatments, they still require work. It's hard to do more of what you love when you're depressed and unmotivated, hard to face your fears when you're fighting back panic, hard to train an overactive mind to rest in the moment. That's where you'll find the power in CBT—to provide not just a goal to work toward, but manageable techniques and a systematic plan to get you there.

In my previous book, *Retrain Your Brain*, I provided a structured seven-week plan to manage anxiety and depression in a workbook format. You'll find this book is similar in its simplified approach as I present the most essential parts of the treatments. But in contrast to *Retrain Your Brain*, this one is designed for those who don't necessarily need to complete a whole workbook. Instead, this book offers a collection of quick and highly accessible research-based techniques that can be used as needed to manage various struggles.

I've designed this book to be useful for those who have never heard of CBT, who are currently working with a therapist, or who have used CBT in the past and want a resource to return to for periodic refreshers. Whatever your prior knowledge of CBT, I hope you will come back to this book as often as necessary. We all need reminders of what keeps us feeling our best.

I do mean *all* of us. I want to assure you that I'm not writing this book from some ivory tower, safely surrounded by abstract theories. Like everyone I'm engaged in the joys and struggles of being alive. I'm excited to provide you with a guide that will truly make understanding CBT simple.

I hope this book is helpful to you so that nothing gets in the way of living a life you love.

CHAPTER ONE

Your CBT Starter Guide

Cognitive behavioral therapy (CBT) has emerged in recent decades as the best-tested approach for managing a wide range of psychological conditions. In this chapter, we'll explore what CBT is, how it was developed, and what makes it so effective. We'll also consider how it can help with specific issues like depression and anxiety.

CBT: The Beginnings

Cognitive behavioral therapy is a solution-focused form of psychotherapy, designed to reduce symptoms and boost well-being as quickly as possible. As the name suggests, CBT includes both a cognitive component, which focuses on changing problematic patterns of thinking, and a behavioral component, which helps develop actions that serve us well. These building blocks of CBT were developed somewhat independently. Let's look at each of these approaches before reviewing how they were joined together.

BEHAVIORAL THERAPY

In the first half of the twentieth century, psychoanalysis was the most common form of talk therapy for psychological conditions. This approach was based on Sigmund Freud's theory of the mind and often involved meeting regularly with a therapist for several years and exploring one's childhood and upbringing.

While countless people benefited from psychoanalysis and similar treatments, other human behavior specialists began looking for ways to provide relief more quickly. They were inspired by recent discoveries about how animals (including humans) learn, and began to apply these principles to treat conditions like anxiety and depression.

These efforts led to the development of behavior therapy by individuals like psychiatrist Joseph Wolpe and psychologist Arnold Lazarus. Wolpe and others found that straightforward changes in one's behavior could bring relief. For example, people with phobias could conquer their fears by gradually facing what scared them. Thanks to these developments, a person no longer had to spend years on a couch excavating childhood events—a few sessions of targeted work could provide lasting relief.

COGNITIVE THERAPY

Not long after the advent of the first behavioral therapies, other mental health specialists proposed a different explanation for psychological struggles. Psychiatrist Aaron T. Beck and psychologist Albert Ellis both put forward the idea that our thoughts have powerful effects on our feelings and behaviors. Accordingly, they posited that our misery arises from our thoughts. For example, it was believed depression was driven by overly negative beliefs about oneself and the world (e.g., "I'm a failure").

According to Beck and other developers of cognitive therapy, treatment first needed to identify the offending thoughts and then work to replace them with ones that are more accurate and help-ful. With practice, people could develop ways of thinking that promote positive feelings and behaviors.

COMBINING BEHAVIORAL AND COGNITIVE THERAPIES

While behavioral and cognitive therapies were developed some-what independently, in practice they are complementary. Indeed, it wasn't long after their development that the two strands were integrated into CBT. Even Aaron T. Beck, the father of cognitive therapy, renamed his signature treatment approach "cogni-tive behavior therapy" in line with the inclusion of behavioral techniques in what was formerly called cognitive therapy. This integration is good news for people in need of treatment and who can now receive a more complete treatment package.

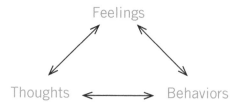

Combining these therapies also helps us see how our thoughts, feelings, and behaviors fit together (see the preceding figure). For example, when we're feeling highly anxious, we tend to have thoughts about danger, and those thoughts will increase our anxiety. These thoughts and feelings in turn will make us more likely to avoid what we fear, which will reinforce our anxiety. Once we understand these connections, it's easier to find ways to feel better.

A THIRD WAVE: MINDFULNESS-BASED THERAPY

In the 1970s, Jon Kabat-Zinn, who was trained as a molecular biologist, began testing a new program called mindfulness-based stress reduction (MBSR), based in practices that have been around for thousands of years. Mindfulness is grounded in the idea that we can relieve suffering by focusing our attention on our experiences in the present moment, as opposed to ruminating on the past or worrying about the future. Mindful awareness also includes a deliberate openness to our reality.

Kabat-Zinn and his colleagues found that MBSR was very effective at reducing distress among people with chronic pain. Since that time, mindfulness-based treatments have been developed and tested for conditions like depression, insomnia, and anxiety.

Just as cognitive and behavioral therapies were joined together, mindfulness-based therapy has been integrated into some CBT programs. For instance, psychologist Zindel Segal and his colleagues found that integrating mindfulness training into cognitive therapy reduced depression relapse once therapy was over. Mindfulness-based treatments are part of what is now called the "third wave" of CBT, having garnered a large amount of support from clinical trials, which is why I've included mindfulness techniques throughout this book.

CBT Principles

Before you begin your CBT journey, let's take a look at some of its core principles. These will help guide you along the path to effective practice.

CBT emphasizes collaboration and active participation. CBT works best when you take an active role in defining treatment goals and deciding how to move toward them. The therapy practice, guided by either a therapist or a resource like this one, brings expertise about general principles and techniques, but it takes collaboration to tailor those components to your specific needs.

CBT is goal oriented and zeroes in on specific problems. A crucial part of the work in CBT is defining the problem, which then makes that problem feel more manageable. Defining clear goals that are important to you is a closely related step in the treatment. These goals will focus your energy and fuel your efforts as we work toward them.

CBT is rooted in the here and now. While some therapies concentrate primarily on childhood events, CBT focuses on how one's thoughts and actions in the present may be a part of ongoing struggles and how changing those patterns might be helpful. Though CBT does consider important learning experiences from early in life, its emphasis on the present makes it an empowering treatment, focusing on factors that are within our control.

CBT aims to teach you how to be your own therapist. With CBT, you'll learn a few basic skills to help you manage the issues that brought you to therapy. By practicing, you can apply these techniques on your own, even with new challenges that arise. CBT is a "teach a person to fish" kind of treatment that stays with you once therapy is over.

CBT emphasizes relapse prevention. Learning how to stay well is an integral part of CBT. By understanding the factors that contributed to your anxiety, depression, or other issues, we can be on the lookout for warning signs of a relapse. For example, a woman who recovered from depression can be aware of a tendency to withdraw from activities that keep her feeling well. These factors are why the relapse rates for depression and anxiety are lower for CBT than for medication. It is critical that a person continues to practice the new habits from CBT, just like someone who learned to play a musical instrument would need to keep practicing and playing to stay sharp.

CBT is time-limited. CBT fulfills its goal of offering relief in a relatively short period of time. For example, a typical treatment program for depression is about 16 sessions; phobias like fear of dogs can be treated effectively in a single session of two to four hours. Shorter treatment programs can also be motivating, providing a sense of urgency to the work.

CBT is structured. Treatment elements in CBT are presented in a predictable order, with later sessions building on earlier ones. Each session follows a consistent routine, too, starting with a review of how practice went between sessions, covering the day's material, and, finally, planning for how to apply that material in one's life in the coming days. This organized approach is a big part of what makes CBT an efficient form of therapy.

CBT helps you address negative automatic thoughts. At the heart of CBT is the recognition that our thoughts often lead us astray. We are prone to negative automatic thoughts, which, as the name suggests, happen spontaneously. CBT helps you learn to identify and respond to these negative automatic thoughts. For example, a man passed over for a promotion might have the negative automatic thought, "I can never catch a break." In CBT, we first learn to recognize what our minds are telling us, since negative automatic thoughts can happen outside our conscious awareness. Then we test the thoughts for accuracy. With practice, we can develop more helpful ways of thinking.

CBT involves a variety of techniques. An impressive array of techniques falls under the CBT heading, from relaxation training to cognitive restructuring to behavioral activation, exposure, and meditation. Part of the work of CBT is figuring out which techniques are most helpful for a specific person. You'll encounter many of these tools in the chapters ahead and will discover which of them will provide you with the most benefit.

I like to organize the techniques of CBT under the headings "Think" (cognitive), "Act" (behavioral), and "Be" (mindfulness). I'll refer to these labels at times throughout this book.

How and Why CBT Works

Most of the principles and practices of CBT probably won't surprise you. For example, facing our fears to overcome them is hardly a novel idea. Those I've treated in my practice are sometimes skeptical that simple techniques like planning specific activities and minding our thoughts can really be helpful. If it were that simple, they reason, they would have gotten better already. As we'll see, CBT is not just about what we do, but also about how we do it. Let's consider aspects of the CBT approach that make it so beneficial.

BREAKING IT DOWN

CBT breaks down big challenges into smaller, more manageable pieces. An overwhelming feeling of depression, for example, can be broken down into a collection of more manageable thoughts, feelings, and behaviors. We can then match specific techniques to each component, such as cognitive restructuring to address depressed thinking. CBT also breaks down insurmountable tasks into a series of doable steps.

STRUCTURED TRAINING

Knowing what we need to do to feel better is helpful but gets us only so far. The systematic and structured training of CBT ensures we get an adequate "dose" of the techniques that can bring

COMMON PSYCHIATRIC MEDICATIONS

The most commonly prescribed medications for depression and anxiety are selective serotonin reuptake inhibitors (SSRIs) and benzodiazepines. SSRIs are typically called "antidepressants," but they can treat anxiety about as well as they treat depression. At high doses they can also treat obsessive-compulsive disorder. Examples include fluoxetine (Prozac), fluvoxamine (Luvox), and sertraline (Zoloft).

Benzodiazepines work quickly to calm the nervous system, acting on the same receptors in the brain as alcohol and barbiturates. Commonly prescribed benzodiazepines include alprazolam (Xanax), lorazepam (Ativan), and clonazepam (Klonopin). In addition to anxiety, they are used to treat insomnia and agitation.

These medications can be as effective as CBT, but relapse tends to be more common if the person stops taking them. Many people benefit from a combination of CBT and psychiatric medication.

Common side effects of SSRIs include nausea or vomiting, weight gain, diarrhea, sleepiness, or sexual problems; benzodiazepine use can lead to nausea, blurred vision, headache, confusion, tiredness, nightmares, or memory impairment, among other possibilities. Prescribing doctors will take into account the potential benefits of an SSRI or benzodiazepine versus the common side effects.

This book focuses on CBT rather than medication. Check with your primary care doctor or a psychiatrist if you're interested in a medication consultation.

relief. For example, we might be aware that our angry thoughts are biased, but when we actually write down the thoughts we're having, we're in a better position to examine them carefully and replace them as needed.

REPEATED PRACTICE

Most of the work in CBT happens outside the therapy office or after the reading we do about CBT. It's not easy to build new habits, especially when we're extremely well practiced in doing things that aren't working for us. It takes repetition to reprogram our automatic responses to difficult situations.

CLINICAL SCIENCE

From the start, CBT has been about evidence and outcomes. *Does it work? How effective is it?* Because the treatment sessions are clearly laid out, CBT programs can be standardized and tested against control groups. Based on these clinical trials, we can have an idea of the average effect a certain number of sessions will have on a particular condition. Recent studies have extended these findings to confirm that CBT can be effective even without a therapist.

Attention! If you are suffering from severe depression, having serious thoughts of hurting yourself, or experiencing other major mental health issues, put down this book and contact a psychologist, psychiatrist, or other health professional. If you're experiencing a psychiatric or medical emergency, call 911 or go to your nearest emergency room. The National Suicide Prevention Lifeline can be reached anytime at 1-800-273-8255.

How Can You Help Yourself?

For CBT to work best, it's necessary to zero in on your particular needs. Are you struggling with low mood, an uncontrolled temper, pervasive worry, or something else? Let's consider how CBT can be used to address different conditions and allow you to help yourself through the particular issues that you are facing.

DEPRESSION

Thoughts, feelings, and behaviors work together in a downward spiral when we're depressed. Low mood and poor motivation make it hard to find pleasure even in things we used to enjoy. We see the world and ourselves in a negative light. As our thoughts and mood darken, we're likely to pull back from many of our activities, further deepening our depression.

CBT can help us break the habit of negative thinking, which can make it easier to get more active. In turn, greater engagement with life lifts our mood and boosts our view of ourselves. If we practice mindfulness, we can further improve our mood as we learn to take our thoughts less seriously. Taken together, these practices can create a "virtuous circle" of mutually reinforcing improvements in our thoughts, feelings, and behaviors.

ANXIETY

When we care about an outcome that's uncertain, the situation is likely to cause us some anxiety. For example, we might be nervous about a first date or about getting to a job interview on time. Low to moderate levels of anxiety are perfectly normal. In fact, anxiety is useful, because being slightly anxious heightens our attention, increases our motivation, and provides us with energy to perform well. Beyond a certain point, though, anxiety becomes counterproductive. For example, excessive social anxiety can interfere with our ability to think on our feet or be present with the person we're talking to.

CBT offers many tools for managing anxiety. Techniques like progressive muscle relaxation and meditation can directly calm an agitated nervous system. Cognitive techniques can address the exaggerated feeling of danger that goes along with anxiety; for example, the belief that others will judge a person harshly if she blushes in class (in the case of social anxiety). Exposure is also a powerful tool to combat anxiety as we face the situations we fear. With repeated practice, the situations become less scary and anxiety provoking.

PANIC

If you've had even one panic attack, you know how awful this type of anxiety feels. Panic is like a fire alarm in your body and brain, sounding the call that *something very bad is about to happen*. Because there's usually no obvious threat—no lion chasing us, no oncoming car swerving into our lane—the mind tends to detect an *internal* threat. *I must be having a heart attack* or *I'm going crazy*. Sometimes you feel like you are about to pass out. Most people with panic disorder will start to fear places where panic is more likely to occur, especially situations that would be hard to escape from, like driving on a bridge or sitting in a movie theater.

Effective CBT for panic includes learning to control one's breath when everything else feels out of control; testing out the panic-related thoughts, like "I'm going to pass out," which often heighten the feeling of danger; and practicing being in progressively more challenging situations so they start to feel more comfortable. With repetition, these techniques can make panic less likely even in situations that used to trigger it. We can also develop a different relationship with our feelings of panic, beginning to see it as no more or less than extreme anxiety, which by itself is not dangerous.

WORRY

If panic is the fire alarm of anxiety, worry is the dripping faucet. Whereas panic strikes all at once, worry slowly grinds away at our sense of peace. When we're prone to worrying, it often doesn't matter what we're facing. Any event can lead to worry, from the important to the trivial. The fundamental question in chronic worry is, "*What if...?*" Frequent worry is often accompanied by muscle tension, irritability, trouble sleeping, and restless agitation. Worry is the core feature of generalized anxiety disorder.

CBT offers several ways to combat excessive worry and tension. We can train ourselves to recognize when we're worrying, which often escapes our awareness. Once we know what the mind is up to, we have more of a say in whether we keep worrying. We can also address some of the beliefs we may have about worry, like that it helps us plan for the future. CBT also offers many ways to "get out of our heads," both through greater engagement in activities and through mindful awareness of our experience. Being grounded in the present releases the mind from its anxious preoccupation with the future. Finally, techniques like relaxation training and meditation can lower the physical tension that often goes along with constant worry.

STRESS

When life's challenges demand a response from us, we can feel a sense of pressure caused by stress. It could be from a family illness, a work deadline, conflict with another person, or any other difficulty we have to face. As with anxiety, a certain amount of stress is helpful, like when a tennis player faces a challenging championship match and rises to the occasion.

Stress provokes a full-body response, as stress hormones like cortisol and adrenaline flood our system and set off a wide range of reactions. Acute stress activates the sympathetic nervous system, preparing our bodies to respond to a threat by fighting, fleeing, or, sometimes, freezing. Our bodies and minds are well equipped to handle brief spikes in stress. However, when the stressors are chronic—like a traffic-filled two-hour commute five days a week, an abusive work environment, or a protracted and contentious divorce—our coping resources get depleted. We may start to get sick more often, become depressed, or show other mental and physical signs of being overwhelmed.

CBT offers tools for calming the nervous system, like specific breathing techniques that dial down our fight-or-flight system. We can also address ways of thinking that amplify stress, such as seeing challenges at work as opportunities to fail rather than to succeed. CBT can encourage us to take our self-care more seriously, as well, to increase our ability to process frequent stress.

ANGER

As with anxiety and stress, anger can be very useful. Anger energizes us to right a wrong, like dealing with injustice. Our anger becomes a problem when we experience it so much that it starts to damage our health and our relationships. Oftentimes our anger arises from beliefs that may or may not be true. For example, was that driver trying to stick it to me when he cut me off or did he simply misjudge the distance between our cars? My belief about his intention will affect my emotional response and whether I retaliate.

CBT offers ways to fix thoughts that drive excessive anger. It can also help find ways to structure your life to reduce anger, like

MOOD DISORDERS BY THE NUMBERS

If you're overwhelmed with anxiety, depression, anger, or other emotions, you're certainly not alone. Among adults in the United States:

- Nearly 29 percent will have an anxiety disorder at some point in their life, including phobias (12 percent), social anxiety disorder (12 percent), generalized anxiety disorder (6 percent), and panic disorder (5 percent).
- As many as 25 percent will experience major depressive disorder during their lifetime.
- In a given year, more than 44 million will experience an anxiety disorder and more than 16 million will experience major depressive disorder.
- Women are 70 percent more likely than men to experience depression and anxiety.
- About 8 percent experience anger so intense it leads to significant problems, with slightly higher rates for men than for women.

starting your morning commute 15 minutes earlier so you're less stressed and impatient behind the wheel. CBT can also help us find ways to express anger constructively rather than destructively.

In the coming chapters, we'll dig into strategies that will help you harness the power of CBT, starting with choosing effective goals in chapter 2.

Getting the Most out of This Book

I've designed this book so you can use as much or as little of it as you need to address your particular issues. Feel free to jump from chapter to chapter to find the set of techniques that works best for you. However, I do recommend that you continue reading through chapter 2, which focuses on goal setting.

I suggest you focus on a small number of techniques as you begin—probably no more than one or two per week. For example, if you're dealing with depression, it is enough for one week to start getting more active. There will be time in the following weeks to address your thought processes, optimize self-care, develop a mindfulness practice, and so forth.

When you do find what applies to you in this book, I encourage you to spend some time with the material and try to internalize the concepts by doing the recommended exercises to reinforce your learning. It's one thing to know what we need to do to feel better and quite another to do it. CBT is about action, and that's where you'll find the real benefit.

Above all, remember that your well-being is worth the investment of time and energy. The work you do now can pay dividends for years to come.

Chapter Summary and Homework

In this chapter, we reviewed the origins of CBT, how it was developed, and what makes it effective in treating depression, anxiety, panic, worry, stress, and anger. The main takeaway is that CBT works by offering structured ways to practice simple and powerful techniques, which is precisely what this book is meant to do.

Speaking of practice, I'll be inviting you at the end of each chapter to do some homework. Don't let the word "homework" scare you, though. CBT homework consists of things you actually want to practice so you can feel better. You're in the driver's seat.

For this week, consider the following questions:

- What is the number one issue you hope this book will help you with?

- What have you tried so far to get some relief?

- What has worked well and what hasn't?

- How does CBT as I've described it compare with what you've tried in the past?

- Finally, how are you feeling after reading the first chapter?

For subsequent chapters, you'll need a journal that's dedicated to your CBT work. If you don't have one already, plan to get one before you start chapter 2.

When you're ready, we'll discuss goal setting in the next chapter.

CHAPTER TWO

Goal Setting

As we saw in the previous chapter, CBT can be helpful for all kinds of conditions. However, before we dive into the application of CBT for specific issues, we need to decide what we want to change. In this chapter, we'll focus on figuring out the goals you want to work toward. Here is an example of a patient and how we worked together to establish the best way to address his needs.

In my first session with Jeff, he told me about the major depression and sleep problems that came on the heels of a long and serious health battle. I learned about Jeff's most important relationships, his family of origin, work history, and other aspects of his life. He was also able to identify a few of his strengths, though he spoke of them in the past tense, almost as if he were talking about someone else.

Once I had a good picture of Jeff's situation, I needed to know what he hoped to get out of therapy. Like everyone else, he wanted to feel better—but what would that look like for him? How would his life be different? What did he want to do more and less of? How would the quality of his relationships improve? In short: what were his goals?

By the end of our first session, Jeff seemed more hopeful. I asked how he was feeling and he said he actually felt a little excited— even inspired—for the first time in as long as he could remember.

By setting goals he had transformed dissatisfaction with his situation into determination to improve it.

Let's consider what was so helpful for Jeff about identifying his goals and how you can develop goals that will inspire your efforts.

The Benefits of Compelling Goals

It's hard to overstate the value of having good goals. When we have a clear vision of where we want to go, it's much easier to commit to the changes we'll need to make to get there. It's a lot like climbing a mountain: When you know where the summit is, you're motivated to keep climbing till you reach it.

Goals also help us stay the course when we run into challenges along the way and compel us to find ways to reach our target. For example, Jeff had been avoiding starting to exercise again because he wasn't sure what he could do given his recent health problems. Once he committed to the goal of exercising three times a week, he started figuring out a program that would work for him. Goals also provide a basis of comparison for how treatment is progressing. Jeff and I often returned to his goals throughout treatment to assess whether we were helping him move toward them.

Goals That Set Us Up for Success

Not all goals are created equal. As you are thinking about your life and the ways anxiety and depression may be affecting things, I recommend keeping these principles in mind as you set your own goals:

BE SPECIFIC

It's hard to tell when you've reached a vague goal like *be more involved with my kids*, whereas *read at least one book per day to my two-year-old* is specific and easy to measure. You should be able to tell when you've met your goals, so be sure to make them as objective as possible.

FIND THE "RIGHT GEAR"

If you make goals too hard you'll feel discouraged, like trying to pedal a bike up a mountain in a gear that's too high, but goals that are too easy are uninspiring, like coasting along in a gear that's too low. Aim for the sweet spot: moderately challenging goals you can reach with sustained effort.

CHOOSE GOALS YOU CARE ABOUT

We'll have little chance of meeting our goals if they aren't important to us. For each goal, think about why it matters to you and how reaching it will improve your life. Along these lines, make sure the goals are actually yours and not just what someone else wants you to do.

Getting from Here to There

The first step toward determining your goals is to understand and accept what you want to change about yourself and your situation. This process requires openness and honesty to willingly face your own limitations.

But first, let's identify your strengths. No matter how much we may be struggling in some areas, we have strengths that keep us going. I often find that the very act of seeking help—whether in

BE REALISTIC

When we've been suffering for a long time, it's understandable that we want to get better as quickly as possible. We might be tempted to try to do everything at once, and set overly ambitious goals for ourselves. If our goals are unrealistic, we set ourselves up for feeling like a failure when we don't reach them. We may start out strong and then fade quickly as we exhaust our already depleted reserves.

As you're setting goals for yourself, aim to balance discipline and compassion, holding yourself to a standard while also being kind to yourself. Sometimes we set goals based on what we're able to do for a day or a week, without really considering what it will take to sustain that level of activity. For example, we might resolve to exercise for an hour, seven days a week, and pull it off for the first few days. But eventually, we won't have the time, energy, or motivation to work out one day. Once the streak is broken, we may be less likely to resume exercising at all.

Part of being compassionate with ourselves is being patient as our recovery unfolds. While it's a worthwhile and inspiring goal to reclaim the life we once had, it's probably unrealistic to think we can get there immediately. Physical therapy is a good metaphor for emotional and mental healing: the right amount of stretching and strengthening may leave us a bit sore for a day, but not so much that we're reinjured or have to stop doing our exercises. So while you're setting your goals, keep in mind that life is a marathon, not a sprint.

person or from a book like this—reflects an inner strength and a refusal to settle for second best. What do you bring to the world? What are your best features or abilities? What do your family members and close friends love about you? Feel free to ask someone who loves you what they consider to be your strengths. Keep these positive qualities in mind as you're developing your goals. In the sections that follow, you'll be considering how things are going in six important life domains. If you have goals related to one of these areas, write them down on a separate piece of paper or in your journal.

RELATIONSHIPS

As a general rule, nothing has a bigger impact on our well-being than our closest relationships. Nothing can really compensate for impoverished connections with others, and we can tolerate just about anything if our relationships are strong and supportive.

If you're in an intimate relationship, consider your relationship with your partner first. If you're currently single and have goals related to finding a partner, like starting to date again, include those goals in your list and return to this list upon developing an intimate relationship.

- What is going well for you and your partner?

- Where do you struggle?

- Do you and your significant other meet each other's needs?

- How is your communication—do you avoid outward conflict at all costs, or is your fighting out of control?

- Are you satisfied with the frequency and quality of your sexual intimacy?

- Do you have enough time together to nourish your connection?

Now think about your other important relationships, including with your children, parents, and friends. Take stock of each connection, and determine anything you'd like to change about the relationship—especially in ways you can control. For example, *I want my partner to be more loving* is less in your control than *I will communicate my needs to my partner.*

As you construct your relationship goals, it may help to consider how your personal struggles with anxiety, anger, or other issues have affected the quality of your connections with others. For example, if depression has led you to interact less with the people close to you, consider setting goals to spend more time with them.

FAITH/MEANING

The good life is a meaningful life—one in which we feel connected to our passions and what we value most. Many of us find meaning through our connections to family. We might also be part of a faith community and feel inspired by sacred texts and a sense of connection to a higher power. Or we may find an expansive feeling of awareness and connection through natural beauty by walking in the woods or in practices like meditation. Whatever the specifics, we tend to find meaning and purpose by connecting to something bigger than ourselves. Think about your own passions:

- What's most important to you in life?

- Do your actions seem purposeful, tied to what you really care about?

- Or do you crave connection to something that really matters?

An exercise that can be helpful is to consider what you'd like the people who know you best to say about you ten years from now. Are there phrases or qualities that come to mind? When Jeff thought about this, he said he wanted people to describe the love he showed to those close to him and the gusto he brought to life—qualities he was having a hard time expressing in the midst of his depression. What would you like your loved ones to say about you? Your answer can help shape your goals in this area.

EDUCATION AND WORK

Work can be a means to satisfy our basic psychological needs. Through work we can feel like we're competent at what we do, whether we're students, employees, or stay-at-home parents. We can also satisfy our need for autonomy through our work if we have some control over what we do and how we do it. Our need for connection to others is also affected by the quality of our relationships at work. How have things been for you at work?

- Do you like what you do, maybe even finding a sense of meaning in your job?

- Has anxiety, depression, or another difficulty made it harder to do your job or interfered with your performance?

- Does your work feel appropriately challenging—not so easy you're coasting along feeling bored, and not so hard that you're overwhelmed by the demands?

Take a moment to write down what you've noticed about your recent relationship to your work.

PHYSICAL HEALTH

There is increasing awareness that the body and mind are intimately connected, with each affecting the other. A psychological state like anxiety can trigger a host of physical reactions (e.g., muscle tension, headache, gastrointestinal distress) and physical states like having low blood sugar can powerfully affect our thoughts and emotions. Let's consider some of the major facets of physical health and goals you may have for any of these areas.

General

You can start thinking about your physical health by focusing on how you generally feel.

- How is your overall health?

- Do you have to manage any major health issues?

- Are there any doctor's appointments you've been putting off?

- Have health problems interfered with your life in any way?

- In general, does your health seem to be improving, getting worse, or staying the same?

Movement

Regular physical activity is good for just about everything. Exercise doesn't have to mean sweating in a gym—any form of movement counts, and the more enjoyable the better.

- Do you get some form of exercise at least a few times a week?

- How does your body feel when you use it—any nagging aches and pains or loss of mobility?

- How does your mood affect your level of activity, and vice versa?

Drugs, Alcohol, or Tobacco

Substances that affect our nervous system influence our emotional state, and our emotions often affect our use of these chemicals.

For example, we might use marijuana or consume more alcohol to cope with work-related stress.

- If you use recreational drugs, alcohol, or tobacco, how would you describe your relationship with these substances?

- Do you often use them to deal with difficult emotions?

- Has your use led to any problems, or does it seem manageable?

- Has anyone tried to get you to cut back or quit?

- Are there any changes you want to make in your pattern of use?

If drug use or alcohol consumption is having a major effect on your life, talk with your doctor about where to find professional help. See also the Resources section at the end of this book (page 188).

Nutrition

The food we put in our bodies can have a big impact on how we feel. These days everyone seems to have their favorite diet—paleo, gluten-free, Whole30, ketogenic, Mediterranean, or South Beach, to name just a few. One thing these diets agree on is that we do our bodies and minds a favor when we eat whole, unprocessed foods, including plenty of vegetables and fruits. We won't feel our best if we eat a lot of sugar, refined carbohydrates, and other highly processed foods.

- Are you satisfied with the kinds of foods you typically eat?

- Has a doctor, nutritionist, or loved one suggested you make any changes?

- Are there changes you've been meaning to make in your nutritional habits?

Sleep

Sleep and emotional health often go hand in hand. Solid, restorative sleep energizes our minds and bodies, while poor sleep does the opposite.

- How would you describe your sleep in general?

- Do you get adequate rest each night, or do you often stay up too late and then rely on caffeine to get you through the day?

- Is there anything that routinely disrupts your sleep, like pets or young children?

- Are you experiencing chronic difficulty falling asleep or sleeping soundly?

- What, if anything, would you like to change about your sleep?

RESPONSIBILITIES AT HOME

Each of us has things to take care of at home, like doing the dishes or mowing the lawn. Think about your domestic tasks.

- Have you fallen behind on anything?

- Are there projects you've been meaning to get to and keep putting off?

- Is anything getting in the way of taking care of things?

RECREATION AND LEISURE

Life isn't just about taking care of our responsibilities. We need downtime to recharge and enjoy the fruits of our labors.

- What are some of your favorite things to do in your free time?

- Do your job and home responsibilities leave you with barely any time to relax?

- Have your mood-related struggles gotten in the way of activities you enjoy?

Make sure you've added to your list any goals for the areas discussed here.

Let's look at Jeff's completed goal list as an example. Notice that some goals, like for exercise, were more specific than others, like finding a better job.

Jeff's completed goal list looked like this:

1 *Get together with friends once a week.*

2 *Get seven to eight hours of sleep per night.*

3 *Exercise four times per week for at least 30 minutes.*

4 *Find a job I'm more excited about.*

5 *Get back to woodworking regularly.*

Don't hesitate to include goals on your own list that will require additional clarification down the road, like *improve my diet*. It's better to have a general placeholder for now than to leave off a goal that's important to you.

It's Not You, It's Your Limbic System

Research over the past few decades has helped us understand the role of the brain in producing our emotions. Scientists have identified a key group of brain structures called the limbic system that underlies emotional experience. The limbic system includes areas like the hippocampus, amygdala, cingulate gyrus, olfactory bulb (involved in the sense of smell), thalamus, and hypothalamus.

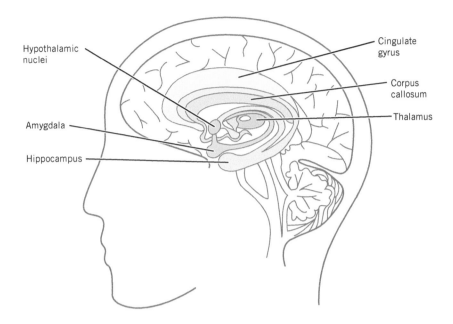

The limbic system plays a key role in activating the body's stress response through the hypothalamus, which controls our hormone system. Thanks to our limbic system, we can feel strong emotions, avoid danger, form new memories, experience pleasure, and many other essential functions.

The limbic system and parts of the prefrontal cortex are believed to have complementary roles, with limbic regions generating emotions and the prefrontal cortex regulating those emotions. For example, activity in the amygdala increases when we're frightened, whereas activity in the prefrontal cortex increases when we try to control our emotions.

At times the limbic system can be out of balance. For example, many psychiatric conditions like posttraumatic stress disorder (PTSD) and major depressive disorder have been linked to overactivity in the amygdala.

It's easy to blame ourselves for our emotional struggles. After all, it's our feelings and our behavior that are affected. At the same time, we often overestimate the control we have over our brain function. When we've gone through a major trauma, for example, we'll likely experience a change in our hippocampus that has nothing to do with our will or our strength of character.

Many factors outside our control can affect our brains and emotions. For example, my colleagues and I at the University of Pennsylvania found that brain activity varied based on genetic differences, current mood, changes in the weather—even poverty, as psychologist Martha Farah's research has shown. Sometimes we're at the mercy of the way our nervous system reacts when provoked.

And yet we're not merely passive recipients of our brain states. Just as experiences outside our control can shape our brains, we can also reshape them based on how we choose to think and act. For example, we can quite literally change the structure of our brains through regular meditation practice. We can also quiet an overactive limbic system and increase activity in key prefrontal cortex regions through certain kinds of therapy.

So there is good news—while we can't choose the brain we're born with or control everything that happens to us, we can use our brains to fix our brains. As you do your CBT work, keep in mind that you are changing your brain.

Chapter Summary and Homework

This chapter focused on setting your goals—what are you working toward with CBT? We reviewed the major life domains, giving you a chance to consider what's going well (including your strengths) and where you'd like to see some improvements. These areas included basic life functions like eating and sleeping, as well as higher-order factors like faith and meaning. Although we went through each area separately, these domains affect each other—for example, getting more sleep can improve our relationships. It should be clear from this chapter that wellness is many faceted, and we need to think holistically about ways to support our best selves.

1   Take a few moments to review what you learned from this chapter. Did you discover anything about yourself and what's important to you?

2   Be sure to write down your goals to make them more salient and easy to remember.

3   Think carefully about the goals you set. Are they inspiring? Specific enough? About the right level of difficulty?

4   I recommend keeping your goals somewhere visible and reviewing them several times over the coming days.

5   Also consider talking about your goals with a supportive loved one, both to get their insight and to provide some accountability for yourself. Simply telling someone our intentions can raise our motivation to follow through.

6   Finally, if you think of any additional goals, add them to your list.

CHAPTER THREE

Activate Behavior

When depression sets in, we often withdraw from many activities due to low energy and a lack of interest. Although this response is understandable, it frequently leads to more severe depression symptoms.

Beth's depression started so subtly she didn't even notice it. She had been very busy between new responsibilities at work and the start of the school year for her kids. Then her mom had gotten sick, which added a layer of stress and additional demands on Beth's time. When she started to feel run down, she backed off her exercise routine to try to conserve energy. She also found it hard to concentrate, so she'd stopped her nightly reading before bedtime, and she rarely got together with her friends anymore. She used to go out to lunch with her coworkers a few times a week, but now she stayed at her desk, declining their invitations.

Occasionally Beth spent a few moments on the weekends sitting outside on her deck watching the trees and the birds, and sometimes she would watch a TV show with her husband. Otherwise Beth's days consisted almost entirely of taking care of her many responsibilities at work, at home, and with her ailing mother.

Depression caused Beth's world to shrink, as it does for so many people. Her mood worsened as she did fewer things for pleasure, and she started to see herself as someone who couldn't handle exercising or getting together with friends. She could still take care of her work activities but found very little joy or pleasure in her life, and felt like she'd aged a decade in the past year. Beth looked forward to feeling better so she could be more active again.

Beth's circumstances were a perfect recipe for depression: being overextended emotionally and having very few enjoyable activities. In order to feel well, we need a balance of enjoyable and important things to do—or in the words of Dr. Aaron T. Beck, we need experiences of "pleasure and mastery."

If we pursue only fun things and neglect our responsibilities, we'll starve ourselves of a sense of accomplishment. On the other hand, we need to balance our work with play. If we're fortunate, we'll have activities that give us both—for example, some people may find cooking doubly rewarding, as both an enjoyable aesthetic experience and an essential task to feed their family.

Why Do We Avoid Activities?

Beth's avoidance makes sense if we consider the short- and long-term consequences of her behavior. For example, when her coworkers invite her to lunch, she thinks about the energy she'll have to muster to make conversation and the possible questions she'll face about how she's doing. It all feels overwhelming, and eating at her desk feels safe and predictable. Each time she closes her office door and eats alone, she feels a sense of relief, which reinforces her pattern of avoidance.

At the same time, Beth is forgetting the positives that come from eating with her work friends. While she might feel awkward at first, in the past she had really enjoyed herself at the group lunches. She would often return to her office feeling energized for the afternoon. She was also missing out on the support her friends would offer.

Invitation to lunch

	Short-Term Effects		Long-Term Effects
Decline →	Relief, low effort	⟶	Isolation, depression
Accept →	Anxiety, high effort	⟶	Enjoyment, support

Two powerful factors drive avoidance of activities:

1 An immediate sense of relief from dodging what we think will be difficult

2 Not experiencing the reward from engaging in the activity, thereby further diminishing our motivation for it

Behavioral activation is designed to break these patterns.

Lead with Action

Like Beth, many of us are waiting to feel better so we can get back to the things we used to enjoy. However, it's much more efficient to gradually start doing rewarding activities, *even if we don't feel like it*. The interest in the activities will follow. This approach is the foundation of behavioral activation for depression.

Think of it like starting an exercise program. At first, you may have very little motivation to go to the gym. Your body may not be used to physical activity, and you might feel more pain than reward from your workout. But if you stick with it, the balance will begin to shift. You'll start to enjoy the exercise high from endorphins. You'll notice you have more energy, which will motivate you to continue. You might start to look forward to seeing your new friends at the gym. If you had waited till you felt like exercising, you might have never started. Behavioral activation works the same way.

"Action seems to follow feeling, but really action and feeling go together; and by regulating the action, which is under the more direct control of the will, we can indirectly regulate the feeling, which is not." —William James (1911)

Strategies for Meeting Goals

In the previous chapter, you identified your important goals. Behavioral activation provides a systematic plan that can be a crucial part of reaching these goals.

Steve had been severely depressed five years ago and had recovered through CBT. Now he was facing many challenges all at once and could feel himself starting to sink into a depression again. He knew it was time to deploy the techniques he'd learned in therapy.

STEP 1: CLARIFY VALUES FOR EACH LIFE DOMAIN

The first step in behavioral activation is to determine what's important to us in the particular domain we're trying to make a change in. What do we value in that area? When we're clear about our values, we're more likely to find rewarding activities that derive from them.

Steve had several goals for his relationships, which had suffered in the past few months. As he thought about these goals, he recognized that showing love to his partner was really important to him. He also valued making his kids feel important and having adventures with friends.

Look at your goals. Which domains do they fall under, and what do you value in each of those areas? You can use the Value and Activities form (page 37) to write down your values in each life area. We'll come up with activities in the next step, so skip those blanks for now.

If you find you're struggling to pinpoint your values, don't get hung up on this step. Feel free to move ahead to step 2 and start coming up with activities. Sometimes it's easier to identify values based on what we like to do. For example, I might realize based on activities I've listed that meeting new people is important to me. Identifying that value can then help me brainstorm other ways of meeting new people.

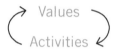

Our values can help us come up with activities that support them, and activities we find rewarding can clue us in to what we value.

VALUES & ACTIVITIES FORM

RELATIONSHIPS

Value: _____

    Activity: _____

    Activity: _____

    Activity: _____

Value: _____

    Activity: _____

    Activity: _____

    Activity: _____

FAITH/MEANING

Value: _____

    Activity: _____

    Activity: _____

    Activity: _____

Value: _____

    Activity: _____

    Activity: _____

    Activity: _____

EDUCATION AND WORK

Value: _____

    Activity: _____

    Activity: _____

    Activity: _____

Value: _____

    Activity: _____

    Activity: _____

    Activity: _____

PHYSICAL HEALTH

Value: _____

    Activity: _____

    Activity: _____

    Activity: _____

Value: _____

    Activity: _____

    Activity: _____

    Activity: _____

RESPONSIBILITIES AT HOME

Value: _____

    Activity: _____

    Activity: _____

    Activity: _____

Value: _____

    Activity: _____

    Activity: _____

    Activity: _____

RECREATION/LEISURE

Value: _____

    Activity: _____

    Activity: _____

    Activity: _____

Value: _____

    Activity: _____

    Activity: _____

    Activity: _____

You can find a copy of this form online at CallistoMediaBooks.com/CBTMadeSimple.

WHAT ARE VALUES IN BEHAVIORAL ACTIVATION?

The word *value* can mean many different things. In behavioral activation, it simply refers to what is important to you—nothing more complicated than that. It helps to divide your values into life areas to make them easier to recognize. Keep in mind that:

- Values have no endpoint and, unlike goals and activities, they continue indefinitely.
- They tend to end in *-ing*. For example, *being* a good friend, *enjoying* time in nature, and *learning* about the world. Conversely, *sign up for a botany class* is an activity with an end.
- Values are often tied closely to our self-concept, as they reflect the kind of person we want to be.
- They can be as grand or as modest as you want them to be.
- Values are personal and vary a lot between individuals.

STEP 2: IDENTIFY LIFE-GIVING ACTIVITIES

Steve thought of ways he used to show love to his partner when he was feeling better—things like rubbing her shoulders in the evening and making her breakfast on the weekend. He started making a list of activities he would like to do more often.

Think of activities that fall under each of the values you identified and add them to the form where you recorded your values. Make sure they're things that have a high probability of bringing you either enjoyment or a sense of accomplishment; otherwise there's no reward. Don't hesitate to list activities you may not be able to do at this point—it's good to have a range of difficulty in your activities, including ones to grow toward. Don't worry if some of your activities feel trivial; every bit of progress counts on the road to recovery.

If you struggled to identify values in step 1, see if your list of activities provides any clues. You can then use the values you identify to come up with additional activities.

Be careful not to downplay the importance of having fun as you're doing behavioral activation. Sometimes we consider our enjoyment frivolous, believing we have more serious things to attend to. In reality, finding joy is serious business and one of the best ways to relieve depression.

STEP 3: RATE THE DIFFICULTY OF EACH ACTIVITY

Some of the activities you wrote down are probably things you're doing already and feel are fairly easy. Others may feel out of reach at this point. Still others will fall between these extremes. I like a simple three-point rating scale for these levels of difficulty—1 for easy, 2 for moderate, and 3 for hard—but feel free to use whatever ratings work for you. The important thing is that the items are rated relative to each other.

Steve found it was easy to take time to play with his kids, while having a date night with his wife would require more effort. He knew he'd have to work up to planning a family weekend getaway, which felt impossibly complicated. Steve rated these activities accordingly:

ACTIVITY	DIFFICULTY
Playing with kids	1
Date night	2
Weekend family getaway	3

Go through your list and assign a rating to each activity. If you find it's hard to decide how difficult something will be, just give it your best guess.

STEP 4: PLAN THE ORDER OF COMPLETION

Now that you have a good idea of how challenging each activity will be, you can plan which ones to start with. You don't have to arrange all the activities in order, but pick at least 5 to 10 that will get you started. That way you'll have a road map to follow over the coming days and you won't lose momentum trying to decide what to do next. You can always make adjustments as you go. Consider including activities from different life areas to provide a variety of rewards.

STEP 5: SCHEDULE ACTIVITIES INTO A CALENDAR

The more specific we are about scheduling and executing our plans, the more likely we are to complete them:

- Pick a time for each activity you intend to do and put it in your calendar. Aim to match the activity with the best time of day for you. For example, scheduling exercise first thing in the morning might work great for a morning person but would not set a night owl up for success.

- Plan at least a day in advance so when you wake up in the morning you'll know what's on your agenda for that day.

- Schedule events further out if they require advance planning, like going on a trip.

- Bigger tasks may need to be broken into smaller steps and scheduled accordingly (see Break Down Big Tasks on page 46).

If you're reluctant to put things in a calendar, consider trying it and seeing how it works. Most of us are more likely to complete a task if we've dedicated a specific time for it. Otherwise it's easy to keep pushing it off.

STEP 6: COMPLETE THE ACTIVITIES

When the time comes for your planned activities, make every effort to follow through with them. It may be especially difficult in the beginning when motivation is still low. Remember that every valued activity you complete brings you closer to your goals.

Before you complete each activity, set an intention to be as fully present for it as possible. For example, if you're at the gym, really be at the gym: see what's around you, feel what you feel, notice what you hear. Let yourself be fully in the experience. This level of presence will help you get the most out of each activity, and has the added benefit of making it harder to get stuck in problematic mind-sets like obsessive worry. We'll address these ideas in more depth in chapter 6.

Applying Behavioral Activation to Your Goals

Behavioral activation is closely tied to achievement of your goals. Let's consider how the structure of this approach relates to the goals you set in chapter 2.

Steve's number one goal was to improve his closest relationships. As he started behavioral activation, he focused on moderately easy activities involving his family members and close friends. In the process, he realized he needed to tend to his own needs in order to be the husband, father, and friend he intended to be. For example, he realized he was more agreeable toward others when he went to the gym a few times a week and ate healthy foods, so Steve added these activities to his list.

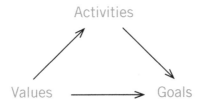

Values give rise to goals, and we reach those goals by planning and completing specific activities. Consider how your own goals relate to your values and activities. How will completing your activities help you meet your goals?

BUILD A GAME PLAN AROUND YOUR GOALS

Behavioral activation offers a step-by-step approach to reach your goals. It's a lot like a team's goal of winning the championship—they'll need a plan for each game to make their goal a reality. Thus, the goals you set will guide the activities you choose and your activities will move you toward your goals. For Steve, *being an involved parent* was a value that gave rise to the goal to *read one book to my two-year-old every day.* To address that goal, he planned the specific activity of *read to my two-year-old every night before bed.*

WORK PROGRESSIVELY TOWARD GOALS

Behavioral activation can bring you closer to your eventual goal by creating a series of increasingly challenging steps. For example, a person might have a goal to exercise 45 minutes a day, five times a week. A workout of that length might be a difficulty level 3 in behavioral activation, so an intermediate activity could be a light 15-minute workout. The success we find in the easier initial steps lays the foundation for more difficult—and rewarding—activities.

THINK HOLISTICALLY

As Steve realized, the areas of our life don't exist in isolation. Just as thoughts, feelings, and behaviors are intimately connected, our life domains intersect:

- Stress from work or relationships disrupts your sleep.

- A friend's unwavering support and concern deepen your sense of meaning and your trust in humanity.

- Struggles with addiction affect nearly every area of a person's life.

- A relaxing weekend increases our productivity at work on Monday.

As you think about activities that will help you move toward your goals, think three-dimensionally. For example, could tending to your domestic responsibilities affect your relationships? Could eating better make you a more productive worker? Progress in different areas of your life is likely to be mutually reinforcing.

Work Through Roadblocks

Behavioral activation is one of the best-supported treatments for depression, in part because it's so simple. And yet that simplicity doesn't make it easy. Even when we intend to follow the previous steps, there will be times we don't complete our plans. When that happens, the number one thing to remember is to be compassionate with yourself. Remember that you're human and that this work is hard.

Part of compassion is understanding how our minds work and creating the conditions that set us up for success. Sure, we can criticize ourselves and try to use sheer force of will to become more active, but there are strategies that can give us greater leverage to complete our plans. Let's consider some of the most effective approaches.

MAKE SURE TASKS ARE REWARDING

A common reason we don't complete our tasks is that they simply don't provide any satisfaction. For example, we might have decided to start running consistently, but in fact we've always hated running. Or maybe we're trying to return to activities we used to enjoy, but our interests have changed.

If you find you're not getting to the tasks you've set for yourself, think about the incentive that you have to do them. Is the activity worth doing, but you haven't been able to muster the motivation for it? Or is your motivation low because the activity isn't right for you? Choose substitute activities if you decide a task just isn't rewarding—for example, maybe you used to love biographies and now you're more drawn to fiction. Go where your heart leads.

BREAK DOWN BIG TASKS

Another common reason we don't follow through on our plans is that they feel daunting. We might be interested in an activity and would find it rewarding, but we can't get ourselves to tackle it.

> Steve had been meaning to do the fall cleanup in his garden, but somehow kept not getting to it. He realized he felt overwhelmed by the job, which by this point had grown to include raking leaves, cutting the grass, clearing out his vegetable beds, and several other tasks. Steve decided to start by making a list of the individual tasks he needed to do, and then he chose just one to get started. He was able to clear out the beds, and once he started working he decided to keep going through several other items on his list.

Momentum is invaluable when we're working to become more active. Like Steve, we can make our tasks small enough to get started, thereby paving the way for continued success. As you review your list of activities, see if any of them need to be broken down into smaller pieces. Use your gut feeling as an indicator—when you imagine doing an activity, do you feel a sense of resistance and dread? If so, break it down to make it more manageable. Don't be afraid to make the pieces as small as it takes to get started. For yard work it might be *find my work boots*. The important thing is finding a way forward, no matter how modest the step.

PLAN ACTIVITIES FOR SPECIFIC TIMES

If you've struggled to complete one of your tasks, make sure you set aside a time to do it. Sometimes we resist making a specific plan because our schedule is uncertain or we like to have flexibility. But sometimes we might have mixed feelings about an activity, and leaving the timing open-ended is a way to give ourselves an out if we don't feel like doing it. By putting the activity in our calendar, we increase our commitment to completing it. It's a good idea to set an alert, too, to remind us when the time comes. Also, do everything you can to prevent scheduling over your plans. Make getting back to life a real priority.

MAKE YOURSELF ACCOUNTABLE

Writing down your plans and putting them in your calendar are ways of increasing accountability to yourself. We can also be accountable to others to provide extra leverage for our follow-through. People I treat often say that having to "report" to me gives them more incentive to complete their homework.

Is there someone you could tell about an activity you've struggled to complete? Choose an accountability partner carefully—ideally it will be someone who encourages you and isn't critical or punitive if you don't complete something. It can also help to have someone who wants to do the activities with you, like going for lunchtime walks with a coworker. Through accountability, you'll encourage one another's consistency.

FOCUS ON COMPLETING
ONE TASK AT A TIME

When we've planned several activities in advance, we might feel overwhelmed by the list. Rather than feeling good about doing our first activity, we might be focused on the other nine still ahead of us. If you find yourself worried about future tasks, remind yourself that the only thing you need to be doing at the time is exactly what you're doing. This singular focus will have another benefit—helping you get the most out of the experience, which will maximize its reward value.

ADDRESS PROBLEMATIC THOUGHTS

As the CBT model makes clear, our behaviors are closely tied to our thoughts and feelings. Certain thoughts can get in the way of doing our planned tasks.

> *Steve caught himself thinking, "Maybe I should just skip the gym this morning—it probably won't make me feel any better." When he thought about it more, he remembered many times when the gym did raise his mood. He decided to do his workout and treat it like an experiment, seeing if it might actually be helpful.*

Other thoughts can minimize the feeling of accomplishment we get from completing a task (e.g., "That easy task was nothing—wait till I get to the hard stuff"), reducing the reward we get from it. Every step in the right direction counts, so treat even the smallest step as an achievement.

If you find your thoughts are interfering with your work in behavioral activation, I encourage you to read chapter 4: Identify and Break Negative Thought Patterns.

Tracking Your Activities

It's a good idea to keep track of how you're spending your time when implementing behavioral activation. You can use the Daily Activities form on pages 50-51. There are several advantages to keeping track of what we do:

- Just paying attention to our schedule can lead us to be more active.

- You'll probably discover some periods of time where you'll be able to add rewarding activities.

- You'll be able to track your progress over the coming weeks.

- You can use the same form for scheduling and recording your valued activities.

Chapter Summary and Homework

This chapter covered the principles of behavioral activation, a simple and highly effective way to reengage with life and lift our mood. It involves a systematic plan for building rewarding activities into our lives, thus making our days more satisfying and enjoyable. We also covered strategies to make behavioral activation work for you when you run into obstacles, which we all are prone to do.

Techniques from subsequent chapters fit well with behavioral activation, such as breaking negative thought patterns, pushing through procrastination, and practicing self-care.

At this point you are prepared to:

1 Track your activities using the Daily Activities form.

2 Follow the six-step plan to build valued activities into your days. It may be enough to do steps 1 through 4 this week, and to schedule activities for the following week.

3 Choose one to two activities to complete per day, starting with the easier ones.

4 Use the strategies offered to raise the odds of following through.

5 Continue choosing activities from your list and scheduling them in your calendar. Check periodically that the activities are aligning with your values.

6 Add activities and values to your list as they occur to you.

7 Have fun! This is for you.

DAILY ACTIVITIES

Today's Date: _____

TIME	ACTIVITY	ENJOYMENT (0–10)	IMPORTANCE (0–10)
5:00–6:00 a.m.			
6:00–7:00 a.m.			
7:00–8:00 a.m.			
8:00–9:00 a.m.			
9:00–10:00 a.m.			
10:00–11:00 a.m.			
11:00 a.m.–noon			
noon–1:00 p.m.			
1:00–2:00 p.m.			
2:00–3:00 p.m.			
3:00–4:00 p.m.			
4:00–5:00 p.m.			

TIME	ACTIVITY	ENJOYMENT (0–10)	IMPORTANCE (0–10)
5:00–6:00 p.m.			
6:00–7:00 p.m.			
7:00–8:00 p.m.			
8:00–9:00 p.m.			
9:00–10:00 p.m.			
10:00–11:00 p.m.			
11:00 p.m.– midnight			
midnight–1:00 a.m.			
1:00–2:00 a.m.			
2:00–3:00 a.m.			
3:00–4:00 a.m.			
4:00–5:00 a.m.			

My Mood Rating for Today (0–10):_____

You can find a copy of this form online at CallistoMediaBooks.com/CBTMadeSimple.

CHAPTER FOUR

Identify and Break Negative Thought Patterns

In the previous chapter, we focused on behavior. Now we turn our attention to another core skill in CBT: tending to our thoughts.

Susan had had a tough year. Her work responsibilities had greatly increased, and around the same time she discovered a profound betrayal in her marriage. As a result, her sleep had been poor for many months and she now felt overwhelmed and depressed.

In her recent performance review meeting, Susan was crushed to hear that her boss thought her performance was slipping. She talked about it with her friend Cathy over their lunch break, and was embarrassed when she began crying. "My home life's a mess, I'm failing at work—I just feel totally inept," Susan said.

As they talked about it, Cathy helped Susan consider aspects of the situation she hadn't considered. For example, she reminded Susan that she had greater work responsibilities because she was so well regarded in her job and had been promoted accordingly. This conversation helped Susan gain a fresh per-spective that boosted her mood.

In this chapter I invite you to be like Susan's friend—but to yourself. You can do this by really listening to what you're telling yourself, which will give you a chance to catch lies and half-truths that have powerful effects on your emotions.

It's much easier to spot the errors in someone else's thinking than in our own. If the roles had been reversed, Susan would have had no problem pointing out how much better Cathy was doing than she thought. We tend to have blind spots with our own think-ing, so I'll introduce a structured approach to monitoring and challenging our negative thought patterns.

The Power of Thoughts

For something that can't be seen, heard, or measured, thoughts have incredible power. Our mood for an entire day can hinge on how we interpret a single disappointment. Thoughts can also have a profound effect on our behavior, affecting whether we forgive or retaliate, engage or withdraw, persevere or give up. No matter what you've been struggling with, chances are that your thoughts have played a role, either in causing your distress or in prolonging it.

In CBT, these distressing thoughts are called negative auto-matic thoughts because they come with no effort on our part. It's as though our minds have minds of their own, and certain triggers will cue these automatic ways of thinking. Just as our thoughts can cause us unnecessary pain, they can also help us heal if we har-ness them to work in our favor. The word *harness* is perfect in this context because it means to control something in order to make use of it. As we'll see in this chapter and the next, we can not only stop our thoughts from tearing us down, but also can use them to build ourselves up.

Let's return to Susan, who's having a rough day. On her rainy drive home from work, she rear-ended the car in front of her. After she sorted things out with the other driver—who was not terribly friendly about it—she sat in her car and did what all of us do when something upsetting happens: she thought about it.

Susan's first thought was, "That's one more thing I've messed up—now they'll raise my insurance rates." And then the image of her friend Cathy came to mind and she wondered what she would tell Cathy if she had caused a fender bender. Susan definitely would not speak to Cathy with the internal voice she directed at herself. She imagined telling her friend, "It was raining and you were in a hurry to get home after a long day at work. You're human. Don't beat yourself up."

Susan felt the frown on her face relax as she looked out her rain-streaked window. "Maybe Cathy was right," she thought. "Maybe I'm doing better than I think." She even smiled to herself a little remembering how grumpy the man she'd rear-ended had been. She felt proud of herself for having kept her composure with him as they exchanged insurance information. She saw that her positivity had caused the man to drop his rough tone. "I guess I handled that all right," she thought to herself as she continued the drive home.

Our thoughts often serve us well, helping us make wise decisions. At other times, our thinking is skewed. Psychologists have demonstrated many biases that are built into the human psyche and these biases can be especially pronounced when we're experiencing extreme emotional states like anger or depression.

For example, I might believe someone is deliberately trying to embarrass me, when in fact their intentions are completely benign. The more often we make these kinds of thinking errors, the more likely we'll experience conditions like severe anxiety. Let's consider a plan for identifying and addressing these errors.

How to Identify Problematic Thoughts

It would be easy to catch our negative thought patterns if they announced themselves: *Hey, here's an overly negative thought— don't take it too seriously.* Unfortunately, we tend to assume our thoughts reflect an impartial take on reality. Ideas like "I am such a disappointment," seem as objective as "The earth is round."

For this reason, we have to be cleverer than our thoughts. Thankfully our minds don't just produce thoughts, they also have the ability to notice and evaluate them. But which thoughts, from our continuous stream of them, should we give attention to?

There are several clues that problematic thoughts may be present:

You feel a sudden shift toward negative emotion. Maybe you suddenly felt dispirited or you experienced a jolt of anxiety. Perhaps you sensed a surge of resentment. If we pay attention at these times, we'll likely discover thoughts that are driving the emotional shift.

You can't seem to shake a negative feeling. Being stuck in an emotional state suggests there are thought patterns maintaining it. For example, you might notice you've been irritable all morning or have been carrying a sense of dread for a lot of the day. Most likely there are thoughts feeding those feelings.

You're struggling to act in line with your goals. Maybe you can't get yourself to follow through on plans you've made or you keep finding reasons not to face your fears. For example, a student might keep putting off writing a paper, driven by the thought, "It's not going to be any good." In contrast, the right thoughts can propel us to action.

THINKING ERRORS

Psychiatrists Aaron T. Beck, David D. Burns, and others have developed lists of thinking errors called "cognitive distortions." Some common ones are summarized below.

THINKING ERROR	DESCRIPTION	EXAMPLE
Black-and-white thinking	Seeing things in extreme terms	"If I do poorly on this exam, I'm a total idiot."
Shoulding	Thinking the way we want things to be is the way they ought to be	"I should have been more patient."
Overgeneralization	Believing that one instance applies to every situation	"I don't know the answer to the first question on this exam, so I'm probably not going to know the answers to any questions."
Catastrophizing	Thinking a situation is much worse than it is	"A customer got really mad at me today, so my boss will probably fire me."
Discounting the positive	Minimizing evidence that contradicts one's negative automatic thoughts	"She said 'yes' when I asked her out only because she felt sorry for me."
Emotional reasoning	Assuming our feelings convey useful information	"My nervousness about flying means there's a good chance my plane will crash."

THINKING ERROR	DESCRIPTION	EXAMPLE
Fortune telling	Making predictions based on scant information	"The rental company probably won't have any cars left."
Mind reading	Assuming we know what someone else is thinking	"They probably thought I looked like an idiot when I couldn't get my slides to load."
Personalization	Thinking events that have nothing to do with us are actually about us	"She seems upset—it's probably because of something I did."
Entitlement	Expecting to reach a certain outcome based on our actions or position	"I deserve to be promoted after working so hard."
Outsourcing happiness	Giving outside factors the final say regarding our emotions	"I can't be happy unless others give me the respect I deserve."
False sense of helplessness	Believing we have less power than we actually do	"There's no point in applying for jobs—nobody's going to hire me."
False sense of responsibility	Believing we have more power than we actually do	"If I were a more interesting speaker, nobody would ever yawn during my talks."

Sometimes the answer will be obvious when we ask ourselves what we're thinking. Other times it won't be immediately apparent. Here are some tips for figuring out what we're thinking:

1 Keep in mind that the thoughts may be about the past, present, or future.

- Past: "I sounded like an idiot."

- Present: "I'm blowing this interview."

- Future: "I'm going to get sick from all this stress."

2 Give yourself the space you need to identify what's on your mind, which might include:

- Finding a quiet place to think for a moment

- Closing your eyes and visualizing what just happened

- Taking a few slow breaths

3 Be aware that thoughts might come as impressions or images rather than words. For example:

- Imagining losing your train of thought and staring blankly at your audience

- Picturing having an accident while driving

- Having a vague sense of being somehow inadequate

Recording Your Thoughts

If you're new to CBT, or it's been a while since you practiced it, I recommend taking some time to record your thoughts and their effects before starting to challenge them. Don't be surprised, though, if you spontaneously begin to adjust your way of thinking simply by being more aware of your thoughts. Our minds have an easier time recognizing things that aren't true once we start to notice the stories we tell ourselves. We usually assume that events cause emotions or actions, skipping over the interpretation we made. In CBT, we work to identify the thoughts between an event and an emotion or a behavior.

When Susan had her disappointing performance review, she was aware of:

Event	Emotion
Critical Review $\longrightarrow$	Sadness

But the review per se didn't have the power to affect her emotionally. Instead it was Susan's interpretation of what the review meant that drove her emotional response:

Event	Thought(s)	Emotion
Critical Review $\longrightarrow$	"I'm messing everything up." $\longrightarrow$	Sadness

The emotion Susan felt makes perfect sense once we know what her thoughts were. We can also examine the link between thoughts and behaviors. For example, we might be trying to get out more but we turned down an invitation to meet up with a friend. This sequence could look like:

Event	Thought(s)	Behavior
Invitation to meet with friend $\longrightarrow$	"I'll probably have nothing to say." $\longrightarrow$	Turn down invitation

When you encounter emotional challenges over the coming days, use this template to record your thoughts. You can find a blank form online at CallistoMediaBooks.com/CBTMadeSimple.

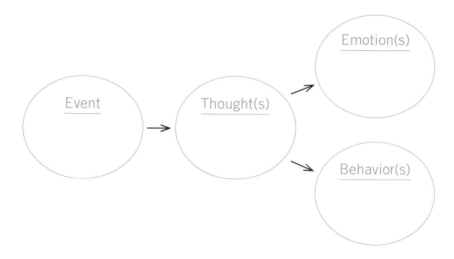

Keep in mind that identifying thoughts takes practice. While we can get better at it quickly, there is always room to grow in seeing what our minds are up to. Our thoughts can have even more power when we consider the CBT model of thoughts, feelings, and behaviors. Recall that each of these components affects the others, such that the feelings and behaviors our thoughts promote will in turn further affect our thoughts. Thus, a single negative thought can be amplified because its effects reverberate through our feelings and behaviors.

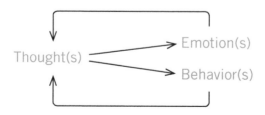

GETTING TO THE BOTTOM OF YOUR THOUGHTS

Sometimes when we think we've identified a negative automatic thought, we're not sure why it's upsetting us. For example, imagine you're getting dressed in the morning and when you look in the mirror you think your shirt looks too small for you. Your mood dips dramatically and you change your outfit. As you realize what's happening, you think back to the event and write down:

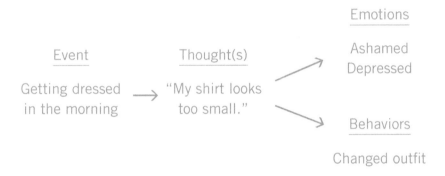

It's hard to understand how this thought led you to feel ashamed of yourself and depressed. Furthermore, there's no apparent error in thinking—you do need a bigger shirt. If there seems to be a mismatch between a thought and its effects, we can use the "downward arrow technique" to look for the actual negative automatic thought. Most likely there is a more upsetting belief that's affecting our feelings and actions.

With the downward arrow technique, we explore the implications of our thoughts—what does it mean? In this example, we would ask what it means that your shirt looks too small. The name of the technique comes from the downward arrows we draw as we trace the line of thinking:

Thought(s)

"My shirt looks too small,"
which means that...

"I've been eating too much,"
which means that...

"I have no discipline,"
which means that...

"I'll never reach my goals."

Notice that with each downward arrow we get to increasingly distressing thoughts, with the last two being truly disheartening. Now it's easier to understand feeling ashamed and depressed. You can use the downward arrow technique whenever you need to dig deeper to identify a negative automatic thought.

Common Themes in Our Thoughts

Different types of thoughts lead to different patterns of emotion and behavior. For example:

THEMES	THOUGHT	FEELING	BEHAVIOR
Hopelessness	"I'll never feel well again."	Depression Worthlessness Inadequacy Loss	Withdrawal
Threat	"I'm going to fail this exam."	Anxiety Danger Uncertainty	Self-protection
Injustice	"She treated me unfairly."	Anxiety Mistreatment Rule violation	Retaliation

The emotions we feel provide an important clue as to the type of thought we had. For example, feeling angry suggests we believe we've been mistreated. Examples of typical thoughts for different conditions include the following examples.

Anxiety	"What if I get sick or hurt and can't work anymore?" "People will see me blushing and think I'm an idiot." "It's dangerous to have a panic attack while driving."
Depression	"I can't do anything right." "I'm letting everyone down." "People would be better off without me."
Anger	"Nobody else pulls their weight around here." "She's treating me like I'm an idiot." "I've been treated very unfairly."

Breaking Negative Thought Patterns

Once you've gotten good at recognizing the thoughts that are tied to negative emotions, it's time to take a closer look at those thoughts.

George is a graduate student in psychology. He taught his first class last semester and was very disappointed to read several negative comments about his teaching in his course evaluations. His impression after reading the evaluations was that most of them were critical. As a result, he began to question his fitness to pursue his dream of becoming a college professor.

However, when he looked through the evaluations a second time, he counted about a 10:1 ratio of positive to negative comments. He also realized most of the negative comments were things he was already aware of and could work to improve, like being a more dynamic presenter. "Maybe there's still hope for my academic career," George thought to himself.

The main strategy to break negative thought patterns is to compare our thoughts to reality. Are we telling ourselves something reasonable, or are our thoughts a poor reflection of the actual situation? Don't worry that you'll have to put on rose-colored glasses and fool yourself into believing things are better than they are. We're just going to see if our thoughts are aligned with the evidence.

FOLLOW THE FACTS

The following series of steps will allow you to identify possible errors in your thinking.

Step 1: Look for evidence that supports your thought

Are there real reasons to believe your negative thoughts? In George's situation, he had a few critical evaluations that supported his thought about being a bad instructor. Take care at this step to be as objective as possible, neither skipping over any available evidence nor filtering the evidence through a negative lens.

Step 2: Look for evidence that does not support your thought

Is there anything your thought ignores, as George ignored the preponderance of positive evaluations? Or maybe you acknowledged this other side of the evidence but downplayed it, just as George knew he also had positive comments but thought it was "just a few" and that they were "just being nice." Counting the number of positive and negative evaluations gave him an objective measure. You might also think about what you would tell a friend in your situation. What would you point out that they might have ignored?

Step 3: Look for possible errors in your thinking

Next, compare your original thought with the evidence you've gathered. Do you find any thinking errors, like those listed on pages 56–57? Notice also if you got the facts right but misinterpreted their meaning. For example, George was right that he needed to improve his teaching, but had catastrophized when he assumed it meant he wasn't cut out to be a professor. So ask yourself whether your thought means what you've assumed. Even if it's true, is it as bad as it seems? Write down any errors you discover.

Step 4: Identify a more accurate and helpful way of seeing the situation

How can you modify your initial thought to make it more consistent with reality? Take care to come up with a thought that is supported by facts, rather than a generic self-affirmation or a simple rebuttal of the automatic thought. For example, George might try to counteract his negative automatic thoughts about his teaching by saying, "I'm actually an amazing teacher," but that thought carries little weight, because it's simply an opinion and not one George really believes. Remember, there's no need to try to trick yourself into better thinking. Simply follow the facts and write down the alternative way of thinking.

Step 5: Notice and record any effects of the new thought on your feelings and behaviors

As we practice new ways of thinking, we'll start to experience changes in our feelings and behaviors. Take note of any effects you're aware of. As always, be honest with yourself, even if that means saying you didn't notice any improvement in your feelings and behaviors. It will be valuable to know what works for you and what doesn't.

The following example illustrates how Kayla, a working mother of four, used this approach when she forgot to call her mom on her 65th birthday.

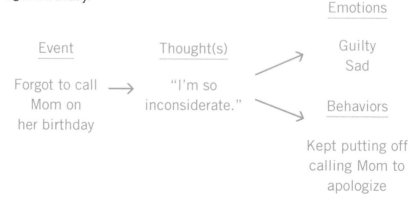

Event — Forgot to call Mom on her birthday → Thought(s) — "I'm so inconsiderate." → Emotions — Guilty, Sad; Behaviors — Kept putting off calling Mom to apologize

Evidence for my thought	Evidence against my thought
• I forgot to call my mom on a special birthday.	• Every other year I've remembered to call my parents on their birthdays.
• I also forgot to send my parents an anniversary card a few years ago.	• I often do nice things for my friends' birthdays.
• I don't always remember my friends' special occasions.	• I was busy taking my sick daughter to the doctor on my mom's birthday.
	• I'm very considerate now of possibly having hurt my mom's feelings.
	• I thought to call her on her birthday but not when I was able to.

Were there any errors in your thinking?

Overgeneralization—I assumed this one mistake defines me as a person

What is a more accurate and helpful way of looking at the situation?

I was busy with work and my daughter's illness, and did intend to call my mother. In the future, I can set reminders to make it harder to forget, but the bottom line is that it's not the end of the world, and my mom was very understanding about it when I finally made the call.

What are the effects of the new thought?

I no longer felt guilty or sad, and it felt good to remember the nice things I do for others.

When starting out, it's best to follow the structure of the written exercise. With practice, we can put aside the formal recording of our thoughts and simply catch and correct our faulty thinking in real time.

Chapter Summary and Homework

This chapter introduced the crucial skills of recognizing and breaking our negative thought patterns. You learned to look for clues and to listen closely to discover what your mind is telling you. You also considered a plan for testing those thoughts against reality.

With practice, you'll probably find recurring themes that show up in your thoughts. These themes are evidence for underlying beliefs that give rise to the negative automatic thoughts, a topic we discuss in the next chapter.

For now, I invite you to take the following action steps:

1 Pay attention for clues that negative automatic thoughts may be at work (e.g., a sudden drop in mood).

2 Practice recording negative automatic thoughts using the form on page 60.

3 Follow the downward arrow technique as needed to drill down to your actual distressing thoughts.

4 Once you feel comfortable with identifying your thoughts, use the five-step plan to start testing them for accuracy.

5 As you gain experience catching and clarifying your thoughts, begin to do so in the moment, without writing things down.

6 Return to the full written technique as needed for more challenging thoughts or to tune up your practice.

Evidence for my thought   Evidence against my thought

_____   _____
_____   _____
_____   _____
_____   _____
_____   _____
_____   _____
_____   _____
_____   _____
_____   _____
_____   _____
_____   _____

Were there any errors in your thinking?

_____
_____
_____

What is a more accurate and helpful way
of looking at the situation?

_____
_____
_____
_____

What are the effects of the new thought?

_____
_____

You can find a copy of this form online at CallistoMediaBooks.com/CBTMadeSimple.

CHAPTER FIVE

Identify and Change Your Core Beliefs

In chapter 4, we looked at ways to discover and change our negative automatic thoughts. If you're new to CBT, I definitely recommend reading chapter 4 before continuing with this one. In this chapter, we are going to explore what drives those negative thoughts. Why do our minds produce those thinking patterns so quickly and effortlessly? We'll delve deeper into the nature of our thought processes and will find there are deep-seated beliefs that underlie our everyday thoughts—and that we can modify through CBT.

> *"Do you mind zipping me up?" Maura asked Simon as they got ready for the holiday party. "There you go," he said as he pulled up the zipper and fastened the clasp above it. Maura turned to inspect her dress in the mirror and Simon thought with a touch of irritation, "A 'thanks' would've been nice." Later, as they were leaving, Simon asked Maura if she wanted him to grab the salad she'd made. "Oh, sure," she replied, and again Simon felt mildly annoyed. It seemed petty to insist she say "please" and "thank*

you," but Simon felt like the small favor he did for Maura wasn't appreciated. He resisted the urge to say a sarcastic, "You're welcome" as he brought the salad to the car.

At other times, Simon feels like his wife doesn't see how hard he works or know how stressful his job is. He sees her as completely absorbed in the lives of their three children, with little time or attention left for him. As he became more aware of these thoughts and feelings, Simon started to see similar sentiments toward his children, as well as at work. One day it occurred to him, "Wait a minute—could it really be everyone else or do I have a tendency to feel taken for granted?"

Simon was beginning to recognize the existence of a core *belief.* Psychologist Judith S. Beck (daughter of Dr. Aaron T. Beck) defines core beliefs as "the most fundamental level of belief; they are global, rigid, and overgeneralized." In other words, core beliefs form the bedrock of how we see the world.

The concept of a core belief captures the idea that *our negative automatic thoughts are not random.* When we pay attention to what our minds are doing, we'll find themes that recur again and again. The specific themes will vary for each of us; our typical responses to triggering situations will reveal our own core beliefs.

A core belief is like a radio station—the songs may differ, but they belong to the same genre: country, jazz, hip-hop, or classical, for example. When you're tuned to a station, you know what kind of songs to expect. In the same way, our core beliefs cue up predictable thoughts. For example, Simon's core belief of being unappreciated triggered negative automatic thoughts about others' lack of gratitude.

By noticing the "tracks" that your mind often plays, you'll discover what frequency you're tuned to. With practice, you can develop the ability to change the station.

Why Do We Have Core Beliefs?

Our brains have to process an incredible amount of information. Imagine you're walking in a big city looking for a restaurant where you're meeting a friend. When you enter the restaurant, your senses will be bombarded with countless stimuli—people standing, others sitting, various rooms, and so forth. If you had to consciously process each stimulus, it would take an enormous amount of time to figure out the setup.

Fortunately, our minds contain "maps" that help us quickly make sense of the situation, assuming it's not the first time we've been in a restaurant. We know the person who greets us is the host, so we explain that we're meeting a friend who will be joining us shortly. We're not the least bit surprised when the host hands us a piece of paper after we sit down, which we know will list the food items and drinks and the price for each. Our entire meal will unfold in a predictable way, through paying the check and saying good-bye to the host on the way out.

This example shows that our brains develop shortcuts based on prior learning. Once we have knowledge about a certain experience, we can navigate it efficiently. This ability shows that we bring organized knowledge to the experience, relying on an internal model that guides our behavior.

Cognitive psychologists call these internal models "schemas" or "scripts." If you pay attention throughout your day, you'll notice many such scripts you follow: getting ready for work, making food, driving a car, and checking out at the grocery store, to name a few. These scripts give rise to automatic responses that often don't even require conscious thought, like when I drive a car safely even while listening to the radio.

In just the same way, our minds develop mental structures that help us deal with potentially emotional situations like rejection, success, failure, and so forth. For example, if we experience a small failure, like missing our train and being late to a meeting, we might think we're irresponsible and respond with feelings of guilt and regret. We might enter the meeting tentatively and with words and a demeanor that suggest not just "I'm sorry" but also, "I've done something bad." These thoughts, feelings, and behaviors emanate from the core belief *I am inadequate*. Being late for the meeting didn't cause that belief so much as confirm it: "See, here's yet another example of how I'm defective."

Maintaining a different core belief would give rise to a very different cluster of responses. If I believe on a fundamental level that I'm a person of worth, I may see my tardiness as regrettable but not indicative of my overall value. I would certainly experience less stress on my commute to work since my worth as a human being doesn't hinge on whether I'm on time. Even if my boss pointed out that I'm late, it wouldn't have a major impact on how I felt about myself.

Sometimes our core beliefs reveal themselves through our assumptions about how others view us. This process is a type of "projection" because we project our beliefs about ourselves onto others. For example, if I make a mistake and assume people think I'm a terrible disappointment, it may be the case that I see myself as a terrible disappointment. Paying attention to what you assume others believe to be true about you can help reveal your core beliefs.

Identifying Your Core Beliefs

Think about the negative automatic thoughts that often come up for you. Do you notice any recurrent messages? You might review some of the common themes that lead to specific emotions and behaviors (e.g., feelings of loss lead to depressive thoughts; chapter 4, page 63).

If you've worked on identifying and changing your automatic thoughts, you can record those thoughts in the outer ring of the figure displayed here.

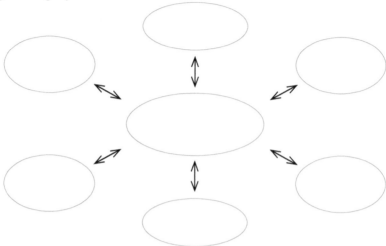

As you consider these automatic thoughts, do you find a central belief that unites them all? If so, write it in the space in the middle. For example:

Esther had a lot of anxiety about her health. She completed the core belief diagram below.

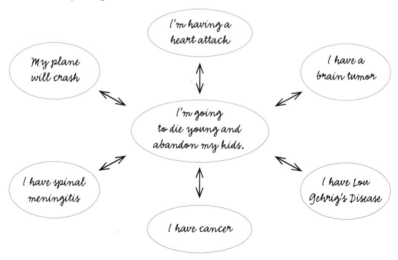

When Esther flew on a plane, for example, she interpreted every bump of turbulence as a sign of an imminent crash. We might expect that many safe landings would weaken her fear of flying since they provide evidence against her fear. However, core beliefs act as a filter that only lets in information that confirms our beliefs. Each time Esther flew, she had automatic thoughts like "We're losing altitude!" that made her think she had narrowly escaped an untimely death. Rather than feeling safer, she was left with the conviction that she might not be so lucky next time.

As Esther learned, core beliefs and automatic thoughts act in a self-perpetuating manner, each being the cause and the consequence of the other. As you become more aware of your own patterns of thinking, be on the lookout for instances when your core beliefs are interfering with an objective take on reality. This process requires paying close attention for the presence of thinking errors in specific situations, taking care not to believe everything our minds tell us.

Keep in mind that negative core beliefs can lie dormant when we're feeling well and emerge when we're gripped by strong emotion. Individuals who are prone to depression are especially likely to show an increase in negative beliefs when they experience a negative mood, raising the risk for future episodes of depression. Thankfully we can train our minds to guard against relapse, as individuals who have used CBT show a smaller increase in negative thinking during low moods.

You can also use the downward arrow technique (see chapter 4, page 62) to get to your core beliefs. At each step, ask yourself what it would mean if your thought were true.

Esther used the downward arrow technique to examine the implications of her automatic thought about having cancer:

Thought(s)

"I have cancer,"
which means that …

"There's no cure,"
which means that …

"I'm going to die soon,"
which means that …

↓

"I'm going to
leave my kids without
a mother."

You can use the downward arrow technique to explore your own core beliefs.

Where Do Our Core Beliefs Come From?

Some of us may be prone to develop negative core beliefs based simply on the genes we inherited. A significant part of the tendency to experience negative emotions—what personality researchers call "neuroticism"—depends on our genes and research has shown that core beliefs are tied to our levels of neuroticism. It's unlikely that genetic differences account for the *specific* core beliefs we hold. These particular beliefs depend on our life experiences.

Sophie constantly battles feelings of being not good enough in some way. She's had this feeling for as long as she can remember and recalls a similar feeling from as early as kindergarten. She had struggled with ADHD as a child, and although she was very bright, had been late learning to read. Her parents had her repeat kindergarten when she moved school districts to give her a chance to catch up with her peers.

Sophie's little sister Claire, in contrast, was reading before age five, and her parents frequently praised Claire for her calm behavior and success in school. As an adult now looking back, Sophie suspects her feelings of inadequacy are based in part on the disappointment she sensed from her parents and her belief that they loved Claire more than they loved her.

A single event of parental disapproval or mild teasing is unlikely to leave a lasting mark. However, a general pattern of treatment will probably shape the way individuals view the world and themselves. If the event is sufficiently traumatic, even a single episode can shape our beliefs. For example, one assault can shift our views on how safe the world is, just as a single betrayal can alter our ability to trust others.

We can also develop core beliefs based on things we observed as we were growing up. For example, if we witnessed our father being constantly stressed out about finances, we may have developed a core belief about economic scarcity. Or if our mother was continually warning us to be careful, we could develop a core belief about the world as a place of constant threat.

Some of the beliefs we developed earlier in life may have made sense at the time but are less useful now. For example, a boy who grew up with an abusive parent might have learned that standing up for himself only led to more abuse. As a result, he developed the core belief *I am helpless*, which reflected the powerlessness of his situation. Decades later this belief may persist, even though he is no longer a helpless child.

Take some time to think about your own history. Are there any events that stand out as possible contributors to your core beliefs? What were the predominant family dynamics as you were growing up? What were you taught earlier in life, intentionally or not? And how might these experiences have affected your views of the world, other people, and yourself? Take some time to write your thoughts in your journal.

Building New Core Beliefs

Once you've identified your core beliefs and written them down in your journal, how do you go about changing them? Let's consider several tools you have at your disposal.

Sophie recognized that her core belief of being fundamentally flawed was probably not entirely accurate. Nevertheless, she couldn't shake the feeling that it was true. As an experiment, Sophie began to look for data that could confirm or disconfirm her negative view of herself. Treating it as an experiment stoked her curiosity—could it be that she'd been making a false assumption all these years?

REVIEWING YOUR HISTORY

Sophie began by reviewing some of her past experiences and was surprised to find at least as much evidence for her strengths as for her flaws. For example, she had managed to get into a good college (even though her high school grades were not stellar) and had graduated magna cum laude.

Sophie found herself discounting her strong college performance by telling herself she did well "only because I worked so hard." When she caught herself using the old negative filter, she realized she'd identified another strength—she was a hard worker.

Think back on your own life history. What evidence supports your core beliefs? Is there evidence that contradicts it? Record your responses in the form. Take care to notice if your core belief might be biasing your memory or your interpretation of events. For example, is a core belief about being a failure making you interpret disappointments as being entirely your fault? As much as possible, make this exercise a fair test of your belief.

As you look over your completed form, can you draw any conclusions about the accuracy of your core belief? Was it based on any thinking errors, such as black-and-white thinking (see pages 56–57)?

Core Belief: _____
_____

Evidence supporting belief: Evidence contradicting belief:
_____   _____
_____   _____
_____   _____
_____   _____

Accuracy of my core belief:
_____
_____
_____

Alternative belief:
_____
_____
_____

You can find a copy of this form online at CallistoMediaBooks.com/CBTMadeSimple.

As with automatic thoughts, see if you can identify a more realistic belief. There's no need to overcompensate and come up with an extremely positive belief like *I'm incredibly competent*, which may not be based in fact and will be hard to believe. Sophie came up with *I have many strengths*, which to her seemed not only positive but reasonable.

Also, don't worry if you have a hard time feeling like your alternative belief is true. Negative core beliefs can be persistent, and modifying them takes time and repetition.

TESTING CURRENT EVIDENCE

We can do a similar test of our negative core belief in the present. Using the same form, you can keep track of the evidence for and against your belief during a day. Look over your sheet at the end of the day and examine the data—how strong is the case for your belief? As always, you don't have to force yourself to believe anything. It will take time to train your thoughts in a new direction.

PRACTICING THE POSITIVE

The negative core beliefs we identify have had countless opportunities to color our thoughts, feelings, and actions. Changing them will take persistent practice, not only in testing their accuracy but also in learning new ways to think. If we only contradict our old beliefs, what replaces them? We need to practice new ways of thinking that will support healthier core beliefs.

Lead with the positive

When we begin to learn how our minds react in certain situations, we can predict our automatic thoughts.

"CYCLING THE PUCK" IN CBT

When I was first learning about CBT, my supervisor was psychologist Dr. Rob DeRubeis, whose seminal work showed that CBT and medication were equally effective in treating depression (you might recognize his name from the foreword to this book). Dr. DeRubeis gave us a metaphor for how thoughts change in CBT that he called "cycling the puck." Hockey players cycle the puck—keep passing to one another while staying in motion—in the offensive zone when they are looking for an opening to score.

The "puck" in CBT is evidence against our core belief, and we cycle the puck by repeatedly considering information that shows our core belief is not true. Scoring a goal means the mind absorbs that evidence and alters its core belief. You'll know the evidence hits home when something clicks mentally, which might feel like an aha moment.

These moments are linked to what Dr. DeRubeis and his colleagues identified as "sudden gains" in CBT, in which depression symptoms show a quick drop in severity. These sudden gains are also linked to a lower likelihood of relapse in the future, suggesting that the cognitive change has a protective effect.

Wendy often gives presentations as part of her job and has recognized that she always expects the audience to think poorly of her. She identified her core belief as "I'm unlikable," which acts as a filter when she presents. Her mind interprets every subtle movement by audience members as evidence that they dislike her. For example, when someone folds their arms, she assumes they're getting impatient with her.

Once Wendy knows what her mind will do when she presents, she doesn't have to wait until her negative automatic thoughts show themselves. Instead she can dictate her response with careful planning. Wendy completed the form below before she gave a presentation.

Situation: Giving a presentation
Relevant Core Belief: I'm unlikable
More Realistic Core Belief: Most people who know me really seem to like me.

LIKELY AUTOMATIC THOUGHTS	RATIONAL RESPONSE
They're bored.	Participants consistently rate my presentations as interesting.
They can tell I know nothing about this topic.	I'm often told my presentations are very informative.
They look confused.	People often compliment the clarity of my presentations.
I'm a lousy presenter.	My boss thinks I'm the best presenter in our division.
They're learning nothing.	People often tell me how much they learned from my talks.

You can find a copy of this form online at CallistoMediaBooks.com/CBTMadeSimple.

Before Wendy gave her last presentation, she reviewed the sheet she'd filled out. She reminded herself of her alternative core belief and read the rational responses to her negative automatic thoughts, pausing after each one to give herself a moment to connect with these accurate observations. As she started to present, she focused on the "plus column," that she gives strong, informative presentations that people enjoy. She also reminded herself not to buy into her core belief if it reared its head.

You can use the form that Wendy used to practice thought patterns that serve you well. Keep in mind that you'll be crafting much more than generic positive affirmations. You'll be generating thoughts specifically tailored to the problematic patterns that have plagued you.

It's especially hard to come up with evidence that contradicts our negative core belief when we most need it—when our negative beliefs are activated and we're being bombarded with negative automatic thoughts. For this reason, it's important to write down the plan for dealing with your anticipated thoughts. It may be most convenient to write your plan on an index card or, as Dr. Judith Beck calls it, a "coping card."

Before you enter a challenging situation, review the evidence for the more realistic core belief. You can even rehearse these more accurate ways of thinking when you wake up in the morning and when you lie down to sleep at night—two occasions when our minds can dwell on negative automatic thoughts. This proactive approach is an alternative to always playing defense and can be an effective means of chipping away at core beliefs rather than reinforcing them.

Keep a record of things that went well

Many studies have shown the benefits of taking stock of positive events in our lives. The practice is simply to write down at the end of each day three things that went well. Next, write down *why* they went well: sheer luck? Something you did? Something another person did? Consistently completing this exercise leads to greater happiness and less depression.

It also presents many opportunities to find evidence against your negative core belief. For example, a woman who believes *I never do anything right* may discover that she successfully resolved a difficult work issue, which contradicts her core belief.

Brush your shoulders off

Once we've identified our negative core belief we'll have a pretty good idea of the types of thoughts it will send our way. With practice, we can take our negative automatic thoughts less seriously. Initially, it's essential to delve into the thoughts, write them down, look for evidence, and so forth—the full approach we covered in chapter 4.

And then we reach a point at which we know with confidence that the automatic thoughts aren't telling the truth. At that point, we can shift to quickly dismissing the thoughts; in effect, giving them the minimal attention they deserve.

Most people find it's helpful to have a set phrase that signals the brush-off to the automatic thoughts. Here are some examples to give you a feel for it. It's important to have one that fits your own voice and style:

- *Oh, you again?*

- *Ha, good one.*

- *Oh, no, you don't.*

- *I'm not falling for that.*

- *What a silly thought!*

- *Funny that I actually used to believe that.*

One caveat: be careful not to adopt a phrase that feels self-critical. We don't want to make this exercise feel punishing.

As we start taking negative thoughts less seriously, we begin to develop a different relationship with our thoughts. The next chapter expands on that notion as we learn about the principles and practices of mindfulness.

Chapter Summary and Homework

In this chapter, we built on the practices from chapter 4 as we identified and challenged core beliefs. We saw how these beliefs do double duty, as they not only lead to negative automatic thoughts but also create a mental filter that can interfere with our ability to evaluate those automatic thoughts objectively. It's not easy to alter our core beliefs, and doing so takes persistent practice. Plan to be patient with yourself as you modify these deeply held beliefs.

The homework for this chapter includes multiple techniques for identifying and changing your core beliefs:

1 Note recurrent themes in your negative automatic thoughts.

2 Use the downward arrow technique to explore the meaning of your automatic thoughts.

3 Review aspects of your past that may have shaped your core beliefs.

4 Test past and current evidence that may or may not support your core beliefs.

5 Practice leading with the positive in situations that are likely to trigger automatic thoughts related to your core beliefs.

6 Keep a daily record of three things that went well, and why.

7 And finally, over time you can shift toward simply shrugging off inaccurate thoughts and continuing on your way.

CHAPTER SIX

Maintain Mindfulness

In this chapter we dive into mindfulness, the "third wave" in CBT alongside cognitive and behavioral practices. Mindfulness has emerged in the past few decades as a powerful way to maintain our equilibrium as we deal with difficult emotions.

Matt didn't know how much more of this he could take. For the past few nights he'd been working to transition his infant daughter to falling asleep in her crib rather than while being rocked, and it wasn't going as smoothly as he'd hoped.

"She should be asleep by now," he thought to himself as his daughter continued to babble away. He had gone into her room once already to resettle her and thought she was close to drifting off when he left. But a minute later he heard her very awake-sounding voice through the baby monitor. A few minutes later her babbles turned to crying. Matt knew he'd have to settle her again.

He shook his head as he entered her room, hoping she couldn't sense his irritation. He looked forward to finally getting to watch his TV show in peace as he patted her back, rolling his eyes and gritting his teeth in the darkness.

What Is Mindfulness?

If you pay attention to what your mind is doing, you'll notice two strong tendencies:

1 **The mind focuses on things other than what is happening right now.** Most of the time we're thinking about events that have already happened or that might happen in the future. Thus our well-being is often affected by things that have little to do with the moment in which we find ourselves.

2 **The mind continually evaluates our reality as good or bad.** It does so based on whether things are working out the way we want them to. We try to cling to circumstances we like and push away those we dislike.

These tendencies are part of what it means to be human. They can also cause us problems and needless suffering. Focusing on the future can lead to worry and anxiety, most often about things that will never happen. Ruminating on events from the past can lead to distress and regret about things that are no longer in our control.

In the process, we miss the once-in-a-lifetime experience that each moment offers. We don't really take in the people around us, the natural beauty of our surroundings, or the sights, sounds, and other sensations that are here right now.

Our constant and automatic effort to judge things as either for us or against us also creates unnecessary pain. We often end up resisting things we don't like, even when such resistance is futile. A perfect example is raging against the weather—no amount of cursing the rain will make it stop, and we'll only frustrate ourselves in the process.

The practice of mindfulness offers an antidote to both of these habits.

PRESENCE

Mindfulness is as simple as bringing our awareness to the present. That's it. If you're walking the dog, pay attention to that experience. If you're having lunch, focus on having lunch. If you're arguing with your partner or embracing afterward, be fully in that experience.

Sometimes when we learn what mindfulness is we say, "I already *know* that I'm walking the dog. I know I'm having lunch. How is that supposed to be helpful?" But mindfulness is more than knowing *that* we're doing something. It's about going deeper, intentionally cultivating a connection with our experience. We don't *just* walk the dog—we notice the color of the sky, the feel of the ground under our feet, the sounds our dog makes, the periodic pulls on the leash. It's opening our awareness to elements of our experience that we normally miss.

At the same time, a mindful approach doesn't require that we do anything in addition to what we're engaging in. If we're running, we're running. If we're driving, we're driving. People sometimes protest that being mindful in certain situations would be distracting, even dangerous. In fact, the opposite is true—we're safer and less distracted when our attention is fixed on what we're doing.

Simply being present in our lives accomplishes two things at once. First, it allows us to get more out of what's happening, so we don't sleepwalk through our lives. We can discover the richness in our reality, even in the most mundane activities. Second, when we're present, we're not ruminating about the past or fearing the future, which is a big part of why mindfulness practice reduces anxiety and depression.

So much of our unhappiness arises from things that have nothing to do with what's real in this moment. For example, I was walking home from the train one evening and started thinking about my children's health. Before I knew it, I was imagining a tragic scenario in which one of them was gravely sick, and I began to feel anxious and downcast as though it were already happening. When I caught myself and came back to the present, I noticed what was real: the lengthening light, the birds flying, the green grass, and blue sky. My kids were healthy as far as I knew. I didn't have to live in my tragic fantasy. It was hard not to smile with that realization as I headed home to see them.

"The way to experience nowness is to realize that this very moment, this very point in your life, is always the occasion."
—*Chögyam Trungpa,* Shambhala: The Sacred Path of the Warrior

ACCEPTANCE

The second core feature of mindful awareness is acceptance, which means opening to our experience as it unfolds.

After a couple miserable nights, Matt realized he needed a new perspective on his daughter's bedtime. The next night he decided to try a different approach—what if he let the night play out however it was going to? It's not like his resistance made things better: it was making him frustrated toward his baby every night. He resolved to do his best to help her fall asleep, and to release his fierce attachment to controlling exactly when that happened.

The first time his daughter began to cry, Matt took a calming breath before going in to her room. Instead of telling himself, "I hate this," or, "This is ridiculous," he thought, "This is what's happening right now." Then he took stock of what that statement actually meant: He was standing by the crib of his baby girl, whom he loved more than words. He was patting her tiny

back, which was the size of his hand. He could hear her breath-
ing begin to slow. He realized how in that moment he had no
real complaint about anything. He wasn't cold, hungry, thirsty, or
in danger. His daughter was healthy. She just wasn't asleep yet.
Maybe things were exactly as they ought to be.

Matt's example reveals important corollaries of mindful acceptance. First, it doesn't mean we stop having preferences for how
things go. Of course, Matt still wanted his baby to fall asleep
quickly and easily, and wanted to have more of the evening to himself to unwind. Accepting meant holding those preferences more
lightly, and not assuming his daughter was doing something wrong
by not being asleep when he wanted her to be.

Accordingly, Matt didn't throw in the towel and stop following
the bedtime routine he and his wife had agreed on to transition
their baby to falling asleep on her own in her crib. He stuck to his
plan, offering predictability and consistency while recognizing
that he couldn't control his daughter's sleep.

When we stop fighting against the way things are, we relieve
an enormous portion of our stress. Earlier in my career I had a
very difficult supervisor, and I often found myself tied up in my
thoughts as I tried to make sense of how unreasonable she was.
Finally, I reached a point of accepting that she could just be difficult, period. My acceptance didn't change her behavior, but it did
free me from acting as if she were doing something surprising. She
was simply being true to form.

A crucial part of acceptance is that it lets us respond appropriately to the facts in front of us. My acceptance of my boss's
temperament made it clear to me that I needed to find work else-
where, which underscores the distinction between acceptance
and apathy.

Benefits of Mindfulness

Training in mindfulness helps with a wide range of conditions. A partial list includes anxiety, attention deficit/hyperactivity disorder (ADHD), chronic pain, depression, eating disorders, excessive anger, insomnia, obsessive-compulsive disorder (OCD), relationship difficulties, smoking cessation, and stress. Many treatment programs have been developed that integrate mindfulness practices into CBT. One of the first was mindfulness-based cognitive therapy (MBCT) for depression, developed by psychologists Zindel Segal, John Teasdale, and Mark Williams. These developers reasoned that the tools of mindfulness were well suited to remedy some of the factors that contribute to depression. For example, practicing paying attention to one's internal experience could strengthen one's ability to detect early warning signs of depression, like unrealistic negative automatic thoughts.

MBCT includes elements of traditional CBT for depression and integrates training in mindfulness to protect against relapse. Much of the training focuses on using mindful awareness to notice problematic thoughts. It also emphasizes learning a different relationship with our thoughts. We can learn to recognize them as simply thoughts rather than something we need to react to.

Multiple studies have shown that MBCT achieves this aim. For example, a study by Teasdale, Segal, Williams, and their colleagues found that among individuals with recurrent depression, MBCT reduced the risk for relapse by nearly half versus the comparison group that received treatments other than MBCT (e.g., antidepressant medication, other types of psychotherapy).

Acceptance and Commitment Therapy (ACT), developed by Steven Hayes, has also received strong research support for treating several conditions like depression, anxiety, and chronic pain. As the name suggests, it emphasizes acceptance of our experience in the service of committing to action that supports our values. Closely related to ACT is Acceptance-Based Behavioral Therapy, designed by Susan Orsillo and Lizabeth Roemer to treat generalized anxiety disorder. And the best-tested treatment for borderline personality disorder—a debilitating and difficult-to-treat condition—includes a strong mindfulness component to address the difficulty handling the strong emotion that is part of this diagnosis. Mindfulness clearly has beneficial effects on many psychological issues. How does this approach lead to improvements?

HOW MINDFULNESS HELPS

There are several ways in which mindfulness practice produces its benefits:

Greater awareness of our thoughts and emotions. When we practice paying attention more and opening to our reality, we begin to know ourselves better. We give ourselves the space required to recognize how we're thinking and feeling and, because we accept reality as it is, we don't deny our own experience.

Better control of our emotions. Greater awareness of our internal experiences helps us interrupt unhelpful trains of thought like rumination and resentment. Adopting a present focus also tends to be calming, which can loosen the grip of runaway emotions.

A different relationship with our thoughts. Our minds are continuously generating thoughts. As we allow these thoughts to come and go during mindfulness practice, we start to give less weight to them. We learn that they are simply ideas created by our minds, and not necessarily a reflection of anything meaningful.

Decreased reactivity. As our relationship with our thoughts evolves, we become less prone to habitual reactions, which are often not in our best interest. Mindfulness can provide a pause before we act on our initial impulse, giving us enough time to choose a response that fits our goals and values.

How Can We Practice Mindfulness?

Like any habit, being more mindful takes practice. There are two major categories of mindfulness practice: activities designed specifically to engage mindful awareness and bringing mindfulness to our ordinary life activities.

FORMAL MINDFULNESS PRACTICES

The most common formal mindfulness technique is sitting meditation. It involves choosing something to focus on for a set amount of time and opening to the experience as it unfolds moment by moment. The most common target of focus is our breath, which is always with us and always happening in the present. Inevitably our attention will drift to other times and places, or we'll start engaging in judgments of how we're doing or whether we like meditating. The practice is simply to return to our intended focus once we realize we've lost it. This focus on coming back to our present moment, without criticizing our minds for wandering, is the essence of meditation.

Other common types of meditation can entail a focus on bodily sensations (body scan meditation), ambient sounds, or wishes of health and contentment toward ourselves and others (loving-kindness meditation).

Formal practices also include more active exercises like yoga and tai chi. In yoga, for example, we can pay attention to the physical sensations of the poses, including the breath that's synchronized with our movement. We can also practice acceptance of the discomfort we sometimes feel in challenging postures, which can lead to either staying in the pose and breathing with the discomfort or changing our position if necessary. Awareness and acceptance promote choice.

"One of the main discoveries of meditation is seeing how we con-tinually run away from the present moment, how we avoid being here just as we are. That's not considered to be a problem; the point is to see it." —Pema Chödrön, The Wisdom of No Escape and the Path of Loving-Kindness

How to Start Meditating

The idea of meditation is simple, but the practice of it typically is not easy. When we sit down to meditate, the mind often decides it has other things to do. Common reactions when we start to medi-tate include:

- Feeling a bit bored

- Feeling frustrated

- Wanting to stop

- Suddenly remembering things you've been meaning to do

- Having countless thoughts clamoring for your attention

None of these experiences means you're doing something wrong or can't meditate, so stick with it. It can help to keep the following things in mind for your meditation practice:

You're not bad at meditating. We'll lose our focus again and again while we meditate. If you think you're bad at it, think again— meditation is simply refinding our focus as many times as we lose it. We don't have to buy into the self-critical thoughts that intrude into our meditation sessions.

The goal is not to "become good at meditating." It's easy to bring the habit of judging to our mindfulness practice, which can make meditation both punishing and disappointing. The point of medi-tation is simply to focus on the present and to let go of judgments.

Let go of attachment to a specific outcome. You probably have expectations of what meditation will be like—having a clear and settled mind, for example—and could strive to make the experience match what you expect. But in reality, we never know what we'll experience during meditation. We can practice opening to whatever happens in a particular session.

There are many ways to meditate. Here's a simple plan to get started:

1 Practice meditation when you're able to stay awake and alert.

2 Find a quiet place where you won't be disturbed, and remove possible distractions like your phone.

3 Choose a comfortable seat on the floor, in a chair, or anywhere else. If you sit on the floor, you can raise your hips with a blanket or a yoga block if that's more comfortable.

4 Close your eyes if you wish, or keep them open and fixed on the floor a few feet in front of you.

5 Practice with or without a recording; set a timer if you do it without. Five minutes is a good starting point. Keep the timer out of sight.

6 Begin to notice the sensations of breathing, paying attention to them for the full length of your inhalation and exhalation.

7 Bring your attention back to the breath each time you realize your mind has wandered.

8 There are many apps and free online meditations available if you prefer a guided meditation. Aura and Insight Timer, for example, are free meditation apps available for iOS and Android systems.

Finally, as with anything else, maintain a light touch. Meditation practice is for you, so beware of making it yet another chore to cross off your list.

Mindfulness in Action

The other category of mindfulness practice happens in the course of our everyday activities. Matt used exactly this approach to change his troubled relationship with his daughter's bedtime. We can bring our attention to whatever we're doing, opening to the experience as much as possible.

Ben loves to cycle around where he lives. It's a very hilly area, so most of the time he's either going up or down a big hill. He realized at some point that he was spending much of his rides hating the inclines, worrying he'd be unable to reach the top of one of the next summits. This had never happened in the 10 years he'd been cycling. He estimated that he spent about half of his time in the saddle preoccupied by the more difficult parts of his rides, which detracted from his enjoyment of the easier parts.

The next time Ben was on his bike, he decided to focus his attention on each part of the ride and develop an interest in the experience rather than resisting it. As he rode, he found he could appreciate the easy parts of the ride more because he wasn't dreading the next hill, and he could allow the climbs to be difficult and challenging but not something to resist. He continued to have anxious thoughts about not being able to make it to the top of a hill but was able to take those thoughts less seriously, recognizing them as just thoughts and not accurate predictions.

As you're practicing mindful awareness in your own daily activities, keep the following principles in mind:

1 Focus your attention on your sensory experiences (sights, sounds, etc.) as well as your thoughts, feelings, and bodily sensations.

2 Open to what is happening in the moment, allowing your experience to be as it is rather than resisting.

3 Bring a "beginner's mind" to the activity, as though it's the first time you've ever done or witnessed it. Let go of preconceived expectations of how it will be.

4 Allow the experience to take as long as it takes, rather than trying to rush through it to the next thing.

5 Notice the urge to grab on to aspects of the experience you like and push away the parts you don't.

6 Allow thoughts to come and go, recognizing that they are just thoughts. Practice neither getting lost in the thoughts nor resisting them, but simply letting them flow.

Mindfulness Myths

Many people have objections to the idea of mindfulness when they first learn about it, and these objections can prevent a person from engaging in the practice. Most of these objections seem to come from misunderstandings about what it means to be mindful. Common myths include:

Mindfulness is a religious or cultish practice. Because mindfulness is an integral part of some religious traditions, we might assume it's an inherently religious activity. However, being in our lives and actually doing what we're doing doesn't belong to any particular religious or spiritual approach, and can be practiced without adherence to any religious tradition (including mystical

BRINGING MINDFUL AWARENESS TO YOUR DAILY ROUTINES

We can focus our attention on anything we're doing. Here are some examples from our everyday activities:

Taking a shower. There are many sensory experiences to pay attention to in the shower, like the feeling of the water on your body, the sound of the water, the warmth and wetness of the air, the sensation of your feet on the stall or tub, and the smell of the soap or shampoo.

Daily grooming. Activities like shaving, combing your hair, or brushing your teeth can feel like tedious chores. But if you've ever been unable to do one of these things, like brushing your teeth after oral surgery, you know the delight you feel to finally do them again. Practice taking your time and doing the activity as if for the very first time.

Being outdoors. Pretend (or realize) you're a visitor on planet Earth. See the sky, feel the air, hear the birds, and witness the trees as if you've never before experienced this strange and awe-inspiring place.

Eating. Notice the food you're eating—its color and aroma, its taste and texture in your mouth, the sensation of chewing and swallowing. Savor the experience as though you've never eaten before.

Reading a book. Notice the feel and smell of the book, its weight, the texture of the pages and their sound as they turn. Be aware of the feeling you have as you settle into a book.

Listening to someone. Notice the person's eyes as he or she speaks, the intonation of his or her voice, the variation in emotion. Practice hearing and seeing this person as if for the first time.

Going to bed. We can end our day by letting go of our past experiences with sleep and opening to whatever this night will bring. Feel your body pressing down into the mattress, and the mattress pressing up to support you. Pay attention to the sensations of your head on the pillow, the blanket or sheet on top of you, sounds in the room and outside of it, the breath moving in and out of your body.

or New Age spirituality). Still, mindfulness is not contradictory to religion. Whatever our beliefs and values, we can embrace them more completely through a mindful approach.

Mindfulness is unscientific. People sometimes object to the concept of mindfulness because they "prefer to live in the realm of fact and science." If you need solid evidence for the benefits of mindfulness, you're in luck—a large and growing number of rigorous studies have found that mindfulness helps with a wide range of conditions like anxiety and depression. It has even been found to change the brain. Mindfulness practice is supported by solid science.

Mindfulness means spending a lot of time in our heads. Language is an imperfect tool, and it's easy to misunderstand what "mindfulness" refers to. Rather than dwelling in our minds, mindfulness is about connecting with our basic experiences and letting go of the stories we wrap them in. To be mindful is to be aware and in a state of openness to what we discover.

Mindfulness means giving up any efforts to affect our world for the better. The word *acceptance* can mean we're not going to try to change something, like when we say, "I've accepted that I'm not going to play professional sports." In the context of mindfulness, acceptance means we don't deny that reality is reality. We're willing to see a situation the way it is. This kind of acceptance can actually be the catalyst for change, as when we accept that there is crushing poverty in our community and decide to take action to ameliorate it.

Mindfulness is weakness. If we assume mindfulness means never taking a stand, it would follow that mindfulness is a sort of milquetoast practice—especially if we equate fighting and resistance with strength. But on the contrary, letting go is difficult. It takes hard work and determination to let go of our habits of perseverating on the past and fearing the future. Mindfulness helps us direct our strength in ways that serve us.

Mindfulness means never having goals. If we're focused on the present and practicing acceptance, how can we set goals or plan for the future? It might seem paradoxical, but planning for the future and setting goals are completely compatible with mindfulness practice. As noted previously, accepting reality can give rise to efforts to change a situation. For example, I might accept that my house is too hot and decide to buy an air conditioner. And we can practice presence even while setting goals or making plans, being immersed in the reality of those forward-looking activities.

Mindfulness equals meditation. The word *mindfulness* often conjures up images of someone sitting cross-legged and meditating, which makes sense as meditation is a very common mindfulness practice. But meditation is not the only way to practice being mindful. An infinite number of activities offer opportunities to develop openness to our experience, from relaxing with friends to running an ultra-marathon. The advantage of formal practice

MINDFULNESS-BASED STRESS REDUCTION (MBSR)

You don't have to be dealing with a psychological disorder to benefit from training in mindfulness. Most of us would be well served by tools to deal with the ordinary stresses of being alive. Jon Kabat-Zinn developed a well-known eight-week program called MBSR, which thousands of people have completed. It includes:

- Education about the principles of mindfulness
- Training in meditation
- Mindful awareness of the body
- Gentle yoga
- Mindfulness in activities

The MBSR program is a reliable way to reduce anxiety and increase one's ability to manage stress. If you're interested in learning more, Dr. Kabat-Zinn details the program in his book *Full Catastrophe Living*. You can also check online for MBSR or mindfulness-based courses near you.

like meditation is that it offers a concentrated dose of training the mind to focus on the now. We can then bring that training into any moment of our lives. Indeed, I've found that practicing meditation leads to more experiences of spontaneous mindful presence in our day-to-day activities.

MINDFUL WALKING

If you're ready to put mindfulness into action, an easy way to get started is to go for a mindful walk. In this exercise you'll practice bringing to your experience greater attention and curiosity than usual. You might choose to notice:

- The solidness of the ground beneath your feet
- The movements and muscle contractions required to balance and walk: the swing of your arms, the push-off of each foot, the contractions in your leg muscles and lower back, etc.
- Sounds you're creating, like your breath and your footfalls
- Surrounding sounds, like birds, cars, and the wind through the trees
- The sights around you, including things you might have passed countless times but never really noticed
- Smells in the air
- The sensation of air on your skin and the warmth of the sun
- The quality of the light—its angle, intensity, the colors it creates
- The particularities of the sky above you

This approach can be applied to any experience you choose, from the most mundane to the most sublime.

Chapter Summary and Homework

In this chapter, we explored the powerful and far-reaching effects of simply being fully in our experience with greater openness. Formal practices like yoga and meditation complement moments of mindfulness in our everyday activities. We also saw how these practices have been integrated with CBT and shown to effectively treat many conditions. If you're working on behavioral activation and/or changing your thoughts, mindfulness principles dovetail perfectly with those practices. Subsequent chapters will include practices from all three pillars of CBT.

It's normal to have misgivings about mindfulness, which often are based on false impressions of what the practice is about. If you're ready to try mindfulness for the first time or want to deepen your practice, I invite you to take the following steps:

1 Begin to notice what your mind is up to during your day. Is it focused on the past, the present, the future? Is it opening to your experience or resisting? Take care to just notice, letting go as much as possible of judging what your mind is doing.

2 Choose a small number of activities to practice mindful awareness during your day, using the six principles presented in this chapter.

3 Begin a meditation practice. If meditation is brand new to you, start with just a few minutes a day. The Resources section at the back of this book provides links to free guided meditations.

4 Reading books on mindfulness can reinforce the concepts from this chapter and contribute to a robust practice; check the Resources section for suggestions to get you started.

5 Practice incorporating the principles of mindfulness into behavioral activation and retraining your thoughts. For example, bring enhanced awareness to your planned activities to maximize the enjoyment and sense of accomplishment.

CHAPTER SEVEN

Stay on Task: Push Through Procrastination

In this chapter, we'll address why we often delay doing what we know we have to do. As we'll see, there are several factors that lead us to procrastinate. Once we understand these factors, we'll consider the many tools that CBT offers for breaking this habit.

Alec knew he needed to start on his final paper, which was due the next day at 5 p.m. "I've still got 24 hours," he thought to himself as he looked at the stack of books he was going to use as references. He felt his stomach tighten with a surge of anxiety as he wondered how the paper would turn out. Just then another video autoplayed on his computer from the "Top Ten Funniest Pet Videos" playlist. "I'll just watch this one. Maybe one more after this one," he said to himself as he turned back to his laptop, feeling vaguely guilty but temporarily relieved.

Do You Have a Procrastination Problem?

People vary in their tendency to procrastinate and in the specific tasks they put off doing. Take some time to consider ways you might delay doing things you know you need to do. Do you find yourself in any of the following situations on a regular basis due to procrastination?

- Realizing you didn't leave yourself enough time to finish a task by the deadline.

- Feeling inadequately prepared for meetings.

- Trying to force yourself to do a task.

- Being stressed about time as you rush to appointments.

- Trying to hide that you haven't been working on a task.

- Producing lower quality work than you're capable of.

- Telling yourself, "I'll take care of that later."

- Waiting to feel more inspired or motivated so you can do a task.

- Finding ways to waste time instead of doing what you need to do.

- Relying on last-minute pressure to complete a task.

Let's begin by considering why we procrastinate and then turn to ways to overcome it.

What Drives Procrastination?

We've all been there—a paper to write, an errand to run, a home project to start, or any number of other tasks we put off. Little good seems to come from these delays—for example, procrastination is associated with worse academic performance and greater sickness. Nevertheless, we often struggle to take care of things in a timely way. The following factors contribute to our tendency to procrastinate:

Fear that it will be unpleasant. When we think about doing a task, our minds often go automatically to the most unenjoyable parts of it. If we imagine cleaning the gutters, we think about wrestling with the ladder. When we consider writing a paper, we dwell on the struggle we'll have at times to express our ideas clearly. The more we imagine these negative aspects, the less incentive we have to get started.

Fear of not doing a good job. We rarely know for sure how something we work on will turn out, and that uncertainty can give rise to fear of doing it badly. For example, when Alec considered writing his paper, he worried that he would have nothing intelligent to say. This fear of possibly disappointing ourselves or others can prevent us from getting started.

Permission-giving thoughts. Sometimes we tell ourselves we deserve a break or convince ourselves we'll work better at some point in the future. In one way or another we justify our procrastination. There are times when these kinds of thoughts make sense—for example, sometimes taking a break really is the best course of action for us. But often these self-statements drive unhealthy habits of avoidance.

Negative reinforcement. Every time we put off a task we think will be unpleasant, we experience a feeling of relief. The brain

IS PROCRASTINATION ALWAYS A BAD THING?

Some researchers have suggested that procrastination's benefits should not be overlooked. For example, procrastinating gives us longer to come up with solutions, and can also allow us to harness the pressure of a deadline to energize our efforts. Management professor Adam Grant cited the benefits of procrastination on creativity in his book *Originals*. According to Dr. Grant, our initial ideas tend to be more traditional. Giving ourselves additional time can lead to more innovative solutions, which we never reach if we finish the task as soon as possible. These potential advantages need to be weighed against the stress, missed deadlines, and poorer quality work that are linked to procrastinating.

interprets that relief as a reward, and we're more likely to repeat an action that led to reward. In this way, our procrastination is reinforced. Psychologists call it "negative reinforcement" because it comes about through *taking away* something seen as aversive. In contrast, positive reinforcement is when *getting* something we like strengthens a behavior—for example, receiving a paycheck reinforces the behavior of doing our job. The negative reinforcement from avoiding a task can be very difficult to overcome.

Is there any task you've been meaning to get to and keep putting off, or that you routinely delay doing? Which of these factors applies to your own procrastination tendencies? In your notebook or journal, write down any ways in which you've been procrastinating and what seems to drive it.

Strategies for Beating Procrastination

Understanding what causes procrastination gives us clues as to how to break out of it. Because there are multiple factors that lead to procrastination, we need a wide range of tools to choose from to overcome it. These tools can be divided into three domains:

- **Think** (cognitive)

- **Act** (behavioral)

- **Be** (mindfulness)

Over time, you can find a set of strategies from these three areas that works well for you.

Some conditions can make procrastination especially likely. Depression saps our energy and motivation, making it hard to take care of things. Individuals with ADHD struggle to meet deadlines due to difficulty focusing on a task and low motivation to complete it. Anxiety disorders can also lead to procrastination—for example, a person might delay writing an e-mail due to fear of saying something stupid. While the strategies presented in this chapter can be useful for anyone, take care to address an underlying diagnosis that might be driving procrastination.

THINK: COGNITIVE STRATEGIES

Much of our procrastination comes from how we think about the task and about our willingness and ability to complete it. Strategic changes in our thinking can weaken procrastination's pull. Refer to chapters 4 and 5 for more specifics about responding to unhelpful thoughts.

Notice permission-giving thoughts that bend the truth

Beware of things we tell ourselves to justify procrastination, or that downplay the amount of time we'll actually spend doing something other than the target task (e.g., "I'll just watch one video first"). When we catch these thoughts, we can treat them like we would any unhelpful automatic thought (see chapter 4).

Remind yourself why you don't want to procrastinate

Putting things off not only can lead to being late or producing poor-quality work, but colors our leisure time with feelings of dread and guilt about the task we're not doing. Remind yourself of these negative consequences when you need motivation to get started.

Beware of "virtuous avoidance"

When we're motivated to avoid a task, we might find other ways to make ourselves feel productive—organizing our cabinets, helping a friend, doing busywork—which can give us the sense that "at least we're doing good things." This belief provides a compelling rationalization that makes procrastination easier.

Decide to start

We often delay doing something because we're not sure exactly how to do it. For example, we might not write a difficult work e-mail because we don't know what we're going to say. In reality, figuring out how to do it is part of the task. Remind yourself that you'll find a way once you resolve to get started.

Acknowledge that you probably won't feel like doing it later, either

We might assume we'll get to a task once we feel like doing it. The truth is, though, that we probably won't want to do it later any

BEING ON TIME

Being late reflects a specific type of procrastination, namely a delay in moving ourselves from one place to another by a deadline. Follow these principles if you want to improve your punctuality:

Be realistic about the time required. Time how long it actually takes to reach your destination. Be sure to factor in time for incidentals like saying good-bye to your family and give yourself a buffer for the unexpected (e.g., traffic delays) so you don't underestimate the actual time required.

Count backward from when you need to be there. Calculate when you need to leave based on how long it takes to reach your destination. For example, if you need to arrive by 6 p.m. and it takes 45 minutes (including your buffer), plan to leave no later than 5:15 p.m.

Set an alarm (with enough time to avoid being late). Avoid losing track of time by setting a reminder, which can also help you relax since you know you'll be prompted when it's time to go.

Be careful about setting your clock or watch ahead to help you be on time. This strategy often backfires because we know our watch is fast and we can end up disregarding it altogether.

Avoid starting an activity close to time to leave. Beware of trying to squeeze in one more activity before leaving for your destination, even if you think it will take "just a minute." There's a good chance it will take more time than you have and end up making you late.

Bring things to do in case you're early. If you're afraid of being early and then wasting time with nothing to do, bring a book or some other enjoyable or productive way to pass the time if you're early.

Combine these strategies with other CBT principles from this chapter to maximize your chances of being on time. For example, use the cognitive technique of reminding yourself how much nicer it is to see your GPS estimating that you'll arrive five minutes early versus five minutes late.

more than we want to do it now. We can stop waiting for a magical time down the road when it's effortless to do the task.

Challenge beliefs about having to do something "perfectly"

We often put off starting a task because we've set unrealistically high standards for how well we must do it. Keep in mind that it doesn't have to be perfect, it just needs to be done.

Choose the Think strategies that resonate with you and write them in your notebook to practice when needed.

ACT: BEHAVIORAL STRATEGIES

The more we rely on sheer willpower to push through procrastination, the less likely we'll break its grip. Rather than trying to muscle our way through, we can find greater leverage to overcome avoidance. Some simple changes in our actions can greatly improve our chances of being productive.

Use external reminders

We can boost our odds of starting a task by making it harder to ignore. Set an alarm, post a note for yourself, write your goal on a whiteboard, or put things where they'll remind you of what you need to do. If you can't do it right away, be sure to set another reminder.

Create a distraction-free zone

It's harder to procrastinate when time wasters aren't readily available. Close your Internet browser if possible, silence or put away your cell phone, and remove any other likely distractions. It's too easy to turn to these things out of habit when feeling anxious (or otherwise uncomfortable) about the task.

Use a calendar

The more specific we are about our plans, the more likely we are to complete them. Put any task you intend to do into your calendar, and do everything you can to protect that time. If you have to bump the task, reschedule it for as soon as possible.

Break down a big task into manageable subtasks

As discussed in chapter 3, breaking down overwhelming tasks can make it much easier to get started. Make the steps as small as necessary to feel doable. Give each subtask its own mini-deadline so you'll know you're on track.

Just get started

Seeing an entire task in front of us can be daunting. Resolve simply to start the task, and to work on it for a short period of time. For example, maybe you take five minutes to outline an e-mail you've needed to write. There's a chance you might even keep working past your modest goal.

Finish a task, even if it's hard

On the other end of the project, keep going when the finish line is in sight. You may as well capitalize on your momentum, rather than having to overcome inertia from a cold start when you come back to finish it later.

Commit to starting a task imperfectly

Procrastination often comes from perfectionism, which can be paralyzing because we can't possibly be perfect. The antidote to perfectionism is embracing imperfection—for example, we can resolve to write an imperfect opening paragraph. This commitment can help us get started, which provides invaluable momentum.

Work next to others who are working

Use the positive social pressure of being around working people to spur you to work. We're less inclined to goof off when those around us are on task.

Use shorter, uninterrupted work sessions

It's easier to get started on a task when we know we'll be working on it for a limited amount of time. Consider trying the Pomodoro technique, created by software developer Francesco Cirillo, in which you do very focused work for 25-minute intervals and take short breaks in between. There are many apps that make it easy to use this approach, though, of course, all you need is a timer. I actually use this approach for all of my writing.

Figure out how to do things

If you discover that a lack of knowledge is feeding your procrastination, add the learning you need as a subtask for what you're working on. For example, if you're not sure how to create a specific type of spreadsheet, plan to watch an online tutorial that covers the topic.

Give yourself small rewards

Use positive reinforcement to overcome the negative reinforcement of procrastination. Research shows that even if we change nothing else, giving ourselves incentives to work significantly changes our behavior. Maybe you give yourself a 15-minute break to do whatever you want after working for 50 minutes, or you get to eat a small treat after every five pages you read. Just be careful that the rewards don't keep you from getting back to the task, like an addictive video game could, for example.

Track your progress

One simple way to reward ourselves is by noting our progress toward a goal. For example, Alec could have made an outline for his paper and crossed off each section as he completed it. The satisfaction of seeing his progress would feed his motivation to keep going.

BE: MINDFULNESS STRATEGIES

The third pillar of CBT offers several strategies for pushing through procrastination, using the principles of presence and acceptance.

Accept discomfort

We often treat discomfort as a reason to delay doing something. But maybe it's not such a bad thing to be uncomfortable in the service of something we care about more than our comfort. If we're willing to open to the discomfort, we can move through it as we get started on our task.

Come into the present

Procrastination is often based on fear of not doing well, which is future-oriented. When we focus our attention on the present, we can let go of worries about our performance and direct our energy toward whatever piece of the task we're working on.

Return to your intended focus

Meditation teaches our minds to return to their intended focus when we realize they've drifted. That same principle applies to our work—if we start to slip into procrastination, we can catch ourselves and come back to what we're working on.

Notice and acknowledge how you work best

Paying attention to what promotes your productivity can lower the odds of procrastination. Notice what actually works for you, rather than what you *wish* worked for you. For example, maybe you like the idea of working from home, but in practice you're never really productive when you do.

BEATING INTERNET-BASED PROCRASTINATION

It was hard enough to overcome procrastination before there was the Internet. As psychologist and ADHD expert Ari Tuckman says, "The Internet just keeps going seamlessly on forever, with links leading to links." He suggests the following ways to prevent online time from sidetracking you:

Accept that you'll probably always want to see one more thing. Internet content is designed intentionally to keep us clicking, watching, and reading, so it's easy to spend more time on it than we intended. There will always be another article to read, video to watch, or social media post to see. Remind yourself that you'll have to step away at some point, and better sooner than later.

Do work before entertainment. If you must work on the computer, do your work before doing things like social media. Otherwise you'll risk spending all your time on unnecessary activities.

Set a timer to interrupt absorption in the Internet. As in other contexts, a timer here has two advantages: reminding you to get back to work and allowing you to enjoy your downtime because you know it's finite.

Don't start using the Internet if you don't have time. It's harder to stop online time than it is to avoid it altogether, so better to not even start if time is short.

MAKING YOUR TO-DO LIST WORK FOR YOU

There are more and less effective ways to use to-do lists. Consider these guidelines from psychologist Ari Tuckman for maximizing their usefulness:

1. **Have a single list.** Multiple lists are redundant and confusing. Create a single master list and give it a place of importance (e.g., a special notebook).

2. **Use it consistently.** A list is only useful if we refer to it as often as we need to.

3. **Put items in your calendar for specific times.** Don't work directly from the list. We're much more likely to do something if we've devoted space to it in our schedule.

4. **Remove items you'll never get to.** If realistically you're never going to do something, it doesn't belong on your to-do list. Save yourself the mental energy and guilt by deleting those tasks, and de-clutter your list.

5. **Update your list regularly.** Rewrite your list to keep it orderly after you've crossed off and added items to it. The time you take to update it will pay off in greater efficiency.

6. **Prioritize items on the list.** By indicating which items are high priority, you can be sure to do those ones first and can relax about not getting to the lower-priority items right away.

Ready to make your own to-do list using these principles? You can use the template below to write down activities you need to complete, including their due date. Then give each task a priority level (e.g., low/medium/high, or 0–10). Finally, schedule a time in your calendar to complete each activity. You can find a copy of this form online at CallistoMediaBooks.com/CBTMadeSimple.

PRIORITY	TASKS	DUE DATE

Chapter Summary and Homework

In this chapter, we considered why we procrastinate, which generally has to do with fear of doing something badly or finding it unpleasant. Negative reinforcement and maladaptive thoughts also lead us to postpone doing our tasks.

The Think Act Be framework presents many strategies for beating procrastination. On their own each of these strategies may have a small effect. For example, research has shown that by itself, rewarding ourselves for productivity provides only a small advantage. By combining these approaches, we increase our odds of success. It will take trial and error to discover what works best for you. With practice, we can develop new habits to replace the ones that promoted procrastination.

If you're determined to push through procrastination, here's a plan to get started:

1 Consider carefully how procrastination is affecting your life.

2 Identify a task you've been meaning to do or one you habitually struggle to do promptly, that you will plan to work on this week.

3 Choose one or two strategies from each of the domains (Think, Act, Be) to help you complete your task. Take care not to choose so many strategies that it becomes unmanageable and counterproductive.

4 Keep track of your progress and what is helpful.

5 Use additional techniques as necessary.

6 Maintain a list of techniques to rely on as needed.

7 Apply what works for you to other areas where you tend to procrastinate.

And, in case it doesn't go without saying, enjoy the greater success and lower stress that come with completing things on time! Congratulate yourself each time you meet a deadline, and notice how much more relaxed you feel when you don't have to fret about unfinished work.

CHAPTER EIGHT

Work Through Worry, Fear, and Anxiety

Overwhelming fear is one of the most crippling emotions. When we're gripped by fear it's hard to focus on anything else, as our nervous system is on high alert and our bodies brace for action. In this chapter, we'll consider the varied manifestations of fear and the tools you'll need to work through them.

> *Kendra noticed herself sighing once again and felt the beginning of a tension headache. All morning she'd been worried about her mom's surgery and thought of checking her phone one more time to see if her dad had called with any news. What if the biopsy revealed her mother had cancer? She was startled a second later when her phone rang, fumbling with it as she answered, "Dad?" She heard the start of a prerecorded credit card offer and made an exasperated sound as she hung up. She felt her head begin to pound.*

Like Kendra, all of us are gripped with fear at some point. We may be prone to frequent worries about things that never happen, or maybe we experience panic attacks when speaking in front of a group. Let's consider a CBT understanding of these experiences.

A WORD ABOUT TERMINOLOGY

Psychologists often distinguish among fear-related words:

- **Fear** happens in the presence of whatever *scares* the person.
- In contrast, **anxiety** involves an *imagined threat* that may or may not materialize.
- **Worry** is a specific type of anxiety in which we repeatedly think about feared outcomes in situations involving *uncertainty*.

For example, we would say that Peter *worried* that he might encounter a dog as he walked to work, felt *anxious* when he saw a dog across the street, and experienced intense *fear* when a large dog ran toward him in the park.

Our everyday use of these words is not as precise, and in this chapter I will adhere more to the common uses of these terms.

What Is Anxiety?

While too much anxiety can be debilitating, too little anxiety is not good, either. We need a certain amount of anxiety to motivate us to take care of things that matter to us.

> Peter was lying in bed, debating whether to hit snooze one more time. He checked the clock—6:09 a.m. His train left in one hour. Peter imagined the consequences of having to take a later one, which would mean being late to his first meeting of the day. His boss definitely would not take that well. Peter sighed, turned off his alarm, and hauled himself out of bed.

Peter was experiencing the right amount of anxiety: enough to get him up and out of bed on time, and not so much that he felt overwhelmed or that it impaired his performance. Like Peter, we have the ability to imagine future outcomes that depend on our actions. Whether it's work, a first date, a job interview, a competitive event, or anything else, we know our actions affect what happens. This knowledge creates a heightened state of energy and motivation to give our best performance. Recall from chapter 1 that CBT looks at the connections among thoughts, feelings, and behaviors. With anxiety, the thoughts are focused on threat, the feelings include nervousness and fear, and the behaviors include efforts to prevent the feared outcomes.

Kendra's experiences with anxiety as she waited for news of her mother looked like this:

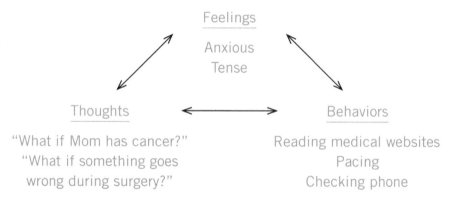

Kendra's worries about her mother's health fuel her anxiety and tension, which in turn cause her more worried thoughts. Her feelings and behaviors similarly interact and reinforce one another, creating a tightly wound state of anxious apprehension.

While Kendra's anxiety manifested as intense worries, there are many ways that anxiety shows up in our lives.

THE OPTIMAL LEVEL OF ANXIETY

More than 100 years ago, animal experimenters Robert
Yerkes and John Dodson provided a clear demonstration of
the link between emotion and motivation. They tested how
quickly mice learned a laboratory task. A wrong answer
resulted in a shock of varying severity. Their results showed
that the lowest levels of shock led to relatively slow learning, as the mice seemed insufficiently motivated by mild
punishment. The highest levels of shock similarly produced
slow learning, as the mice seemed to have reached a
heightened state of arousal that interfered with learning.

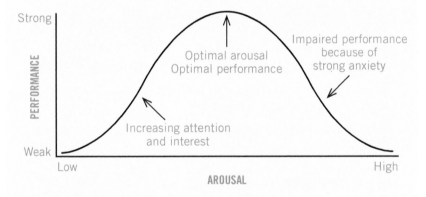

Psychologists call this pattern an "inverted U" because of
the shape it makes when graphed.

Humans show the same inverted U pattern as a function of
their anxiety; too little and too much hurt our performance,
and modest amounts maximize our success. For example,
moderate amounts of stimulants like coffee can increase
our energy and focus, while higher amounts make us feel
jittery and overstimulated.

The Many Faces of Fear

Anxiety disorders are the most common psychiatric diagnoses, encompassing a wide range of conditions. In their most recent revision, the creators of the *Diagnostic and Statistical Manual of Mental Disorders*, 5th edition (*DSM-5*) removed OCD and PTSD from the anxiety disorders, placing each one in its own category. There were various reasons for these changes, but it remains widely understood that both of these conditions can feature a strong dose of anxiety. PTSD and OCD also respond to similar treatment approaches as the remaining anxiety disorders, and so they are included in this chapter.

SPECIFIC PHOBIA

Excessive fear of certain stimuli may indicate a specific phobia. The person may realize their fears are overblown, which doesn't make it any easier to shake them. Avoidance of the feared object or situation is very common.

Anything can become an object of fear, but certain ones are most typical. They include:

- **Certain situations** (e.g., riding in an elevator, flying in an airplane)

- **Natural environments** (e.g., thunderstorms, heights)

- **Animals** (e.g., spiders, snakes)

- **Blood-injection-injury** (e.g., giving blood, getting a shot)

SOCIAL ANXIETY DISORDER

It's normal to feel a moderate amount of anxiety in social situations, especially when we're performing or being evaluated. Social anxiety may be a disorder when it's so strong that it causes tremendous distress or leads a person to avoid situations that would trigger it. Typical feared situations include:

- Giving a speech or presentation
- Talking in a group of people
- Eating in front of others
- Going to a party
- Being the center of attention
- Disagreeing with someone
- Meeting new people

In each of these situations, the person is afraid of doing something embarrassing or otherwise having others think badly of them. Part of what can make social anxiety persist is that it's hard to disconfirm the fears. How do we know, for example, that people didn't hate our wedding speech, even if they do the socially expected thing and tell us it was great? The uncertainty inherent in social situations can perpetuate our fears.

PANIC DISORDER

A panic attack is a discrete spell of intense anxiety, usually accompanied by physical symptoms like sweating, pounding heart, and shortness of breath. Panic often involves alterations in our sense of reality, such as feeling like things aren't real (derealization) or feeling detached from our experience (depersonalization).

Most people will have at least one panic attack in their lives. Panic is part of a disorder when it leads to fear that something terrible is happening (e.g., "I'm having a stroke") or when a person has intense dread of the next attack.

Panic attacks are so aversive that people with panic disorder often begin to avoid any situation where they're liable to panic, especially if it would be difficult to escape. Common situations people avoid include bridges, movie theaters (especially sitting in the middle of a row), and trains. This type of avoidance may warrant an additional diagnosis of agoraphobia.

"Part of being human is managing the balance between anticipating the future and accepting its uncertainty. Worry is a sign that the balance has been disrupted." —Susan M. Orsillo and Lizabeth Roemer, The Mindful Way Through Anxiety

GENERALIZED ANXIETY DISORDER (GAD)

While panic disorder represents the sense of immediate danger, GAD involves a more diffuse anxiety about future events. The core of GAD is continual worry about a wide range of things (as "generalized" suggests). Someone I know likened GAD to the stress of final exam week but applied to every situation in one's life. The excessive and uncontrollable worry in GAD leads to symptoms like difficulty concentrating, trouble sleeping, muscle tension, and restlessness.

POSTTRAUMATIC STRESS DISORDER (PTSD)

Anxiety is an understandable response when we've been through a terrible traumatic event. Anything that poses a threat to our physical well-being can lead to PTSD, including natural disasters, car accidents, muggings, sexual assaults, and combat, among others. Witnessing something awful happen to someone else or learning about a trauma that someone close to us experienced can also set us up for PTSD.

After experiencing a terrible trauma, most people will have symptoms like:

1 **Reimagining and reexperiencing.** This includes intrusive memories, nightmares, and strong emotional reactions when reminded of the event.

2 **Avoidance.** This includes trying not to think about the trauma, as well as avoiding people, places, and things that remind the person of what happened.

3 **Changes in thinking and mood**. For example, we may start to see the world as a very dangerous place and ourselves as powerless to cope with it. We might also struggle to trust others, and paradoxically begin to engage in risky behaviors. We're also less likely to experience positive emotions and more likely to experience negative ones.

4 **Hyperarousal.** This means our nervous systems are on high alert. We may have trouble sleeping and concentrating, and may constantly be checking our surroundings for danger.

These reactions are very typical for nearly everyone after a trauma. To meet PTSD criteria, they have to meet the somewhat arbitrary criterion of lasting more than one month.

OBSESSIVE-COMPULSIVE DISORDER (OCD)

Our brains are wired to detect the possibility of danger and try to avoid it. A glitch in this essential function can lead to OCD. The **obsessions** in OCD are repetitive thoughts about something bad that might happen, like getting sick, offending God, causing a fire, or harming another person. Naturally a person wants to avoid these feared outcomes, which leads to the irresistible urge to neutralize the obsessive fear through **compulsions**.

Examples of the obsession–compulsion cycle include:

Fear of getting sick → Wash hands

Fear of having hit a pedestrian → Check the rearview mirror

Fear of having committed blasphemy → Say a ritualized prayer

The compulsions are powerfully reinforcing through the negative reinforcement discussed in chapter 7 (see page 106). At the same time, people with OCD usually still feel uneasy after doing the compulsion, because there is no way to know for sure that what they fear won't happen. As a result, a person with OCD is likely to repeat the compulsion and can spend hours a day stuck in the obsession–compulsion cycle.

While many conditions will improve with various kinds of psychotherapy, OCD requires a specific treatment. The best-tested therapy is called exposure and response prevention, which is a type of CBT. As the name indicates, it involves exposing oneself to the OCD-related fears and giving up the compulsions that maintain the disorder. Check the Resources section of this book if you're looking for effective OCD treatment.

OTHER MANIFESTATIONS

Even if you don't meet criteria for any of these *DSM-5* anxiety conditions, fear can still play an unhelpful role in your life. For example, the subtle and consistent ways in which we make decisions based on fear can have profound effects on the course of our lives. What's more, these manifestations of fear can be so pervasive we don't even recognize them. These are the fears that keep us stuck not in a debilitating disorder but in a life half-lived.

You can see these kinds of fears at work in:

- Holding ourselves back out of fear of success

- Avoiding taking reasonable risks out of fear of failure

- Living the way we think others expect us to and not how we want to live

- Avoiding the vulnerability that comes with true intimacy

- Experiencing anger that arises from fear (e.g., being mad at a loved one for being late because we worried for their safety)

Take some time to consider how fear shows up in your own life. While fear is designed to keep us safe, it can keep us from living freely and fully if we let it guide our actions.

Let's turn now to the tools that can help relieve anxiety.

Strategies for Working Through Worry, Fear, and Anxiety

There are many tools for managing overwhelming worry, fear, and anxiety, including cognitive, behavioral, and mindfulness techniques.

THINK (COGNITIVE)

When our fear is activated, we're likely to have thoughts that terrify us even more. For example, if we're gripped by fear on a plane, we might become convinced the plane is going to crash, which further heightens our fear and continues the cycle (refer to the CBT

ANXIETY AND YOUR BRAIN

Imagine you're enjoying a nice walk through the woods when you encounter a slithery thing on the ground. Light that's reflected off the object will enter your eyes and fall on your retinas, leading to signals that travel through the brain's relay station (the thalamus) and into the primary visual areas located at the back of your brain. The information is then relayed to other parts of the brain, including memory areas that match the object with the concept "snake."

The fact that you're seeing a snake is then passed along to other areas, including the amygdala, tucked deep inside your brain, which is central to feeling and expressing fear and other emotions. How does your brain know to fear a snake next to your foot on the ground but not the one behind the glass at the zoo? The amygdala also gets input from the hippocampus, which is crucial for understanding context. Thanks to your hippocampus you may even start to feel afraid the next time you walk through the woods, even if you don't run into a snake.

Signals from the amygdala then activate a brain area called the hypothalamus, which will activate the fight-or-flight response of the sympathetic nervous system through the release of stress hormones like epinephrine (adrenaline). The hypothalamus also triggers the pituitary gland to release hormones into your bloodstream that travel to your adrenal glands (which sit on top of your kidneys), causing them to release additional stress hormones like cortisol. Our existence on this planet has depended on this coordinated response, allowing us to recognize and respond to threats, like moving away from the snake.

Just as it's important for our survival to learn to fear certain stimuli, it is also adaptive to learn when danger is minimal so we're not overly fearful. This new learning depends on providing our brains with new information, which anxiety-driven avoidance can prevent. For example, if I always avoid dogs because a big dog knocked me down when I was a little kid, I'll never learn that my early encounter won't be my typical experience with dogs. When we practice mindfulness and cognitive behavioral techniques for dealing with fear and anxiety, we are retraining these brain areas to change their response to things that scare us.

model of anxiety at the beginning of this chapter). By challenging our anxious thoughts, we can interrupt this feedback loop.

A note of caution: when we're overwhelmed with anxiety, it's difficult or even impossible to talk ourselves down with reason alone. These techniques will tend to be most effective before anxiety has taken over and in combination with behavioral and mindfulness techniques.

Remember that anxiety is not dangerous. We often come to fear anxiety itself, believing it's dangerous to be too anxious. However, as uncomfortable as it can be, anxiety itself is not harmful. Furthermore, fear about being anxious only leads to more anxiety. Keep in mind even in a severe bout of anxiety that the physical, mental, and emotional symptoms will not hurt you.

Reassess the likelihood of danger. Our fear will convince us that what we're afraid of is really going to happen. But keep in mind that anxiety disorders by definition involve unrealistic fears given the actual risk, so the probability that they will come true is actually quite low. If your fear is telling you something really bad is likely to happen, you can use the Core Belief form from chapter 5 (see page 79) to test this belief. How strong is the evidence supporting it? Is there any evidence against it? Has it happened before, and if so, with what frequency? If you discover any errors in your thinking, reevaluate the likelihood that what you fear will actually happen in light of the evidence.

Reassess the severity of threat. Sometimes the thinking error we make isn't about how *likely* a negative outcome is but how *bad* it would be. For example, Joe thought it would be terrible if people knew he was anxious while giving a talk. As he examined this thought, he realized that people might indeed know he was anxious from the quaver in his voice or his shaking hands, but realized it probably wouldn't be a big deal. After all, he'd heard speakers who seemed nervous before, and their anxiety hadn't colored his overall perception of the person or the quality of his or her speech.

Why worry? Worrying is a hard habit to break, especially because we often believe we *should* worry. We might tell ourselves that worrying:

- Helps us think of solutions to a problem

- Prevents us from being blindsided by bad news

- Shows we care

- Can make things turn out well

- Helps motivate us

These beliefs generally are false. For example, we can't avoid potential pain by imagining the worst-case scenario, which would be just as upsetting if it actually happened—plus we feel needless distress from countless worries that never materialize. When we see the futility of worry, we're more likely to redirect our thoughts.

Test your predictions. This technique sits at the intersection of cognitive and behavioral approaches. When you've identified a fear about how a specific situation will turn out, you can design a way to see if your forecast was right.

Lily dealt with a lot of social anxiety at work. She was convinced that if she spoke up in a meeting, her colleagues would ignore her ideas and probably even criticize them. She wrote down these and other expected outcomes before a meeting, and then she took a risk and volunteered her thoughts. While people seemed a bit surprised when she spoke up, nobody criticized her ideas. In fact, her supervisor asked her to lead a subgroup that would develop her proposal. After the meeting, Lily wrote down the actual outcome versus her prediction.

As we saw in chapter 5, our core beliefs can distort our memories, thereby reinforcing our beliefs. It's important to record when our predictions turn out to be false, to help us encode and remember information that's counter to our expectations. Testing our predictions is closely tied to exposure, which we'll explore later in this chapter.

ACT (BEHAVIORAL)

When we change how we respond to situations that make us anxious, we can learn new behaviors that lessen our fear. Let's review some strategies for using our actions to combat our anxiety.

Approach what you fear. Facing our fears head-on is called "exposure therapy" in CBT and is the antidote to the avoidance that maintains anxiety. (This assumes, of course, that what we fear is not actually very risky; facing a dog that bites won't fix our phobia of animals, for example.) Exposure to the things that scare us decreases our anxiety by:

- Allowing our nervous system to learn that the danger is exaggerated

- Giving us confidence that we can face our fears without being overwhelmed

- Reinforcing our awareness that anxiety is not dangerous

Hundreds of studies have found that exposure is a powerful weapon against overblown anxiety; later in this chapter we'll go through a step-by-step plan for implementing exposure.

Face your physical manifestations of fear. Anxiety about our anxiety can present an additional challenge. Panic disorder in particular can feature a fear of the panic-related physical sensations. For example, a person might avoid running because the resulting shortness of breath and pounding heart are similar to the feelings during panic. Avoiding physical sensations only strengthens our fear and makes us more sensitive to the sensations. Exposure therapy can decrease our fear of physical anxiety symptoms. For example, we can do jumping jacks to cause breathlessness, spin in a chair to induce dizziness, or wear warm clothes to make ourselves sweat. Doing these kinds of things repeatedly lessens our fear of the physical sensations.

Let go of safety behaviors. When we have to do something that scares us, we often incorporate behaviors that are intended to prevent what we're afraid of from happening. For example, if we're afraid of going blank while giving a talk, we might write out and read our whole presentation. Other examples include:

- Keeping our hands in our pockets in social situations in case our hands shake

- Being overly cautious to avoid offending anyone

- Traveling with a companion only because of anxiety

- Triple-checking an e-mail for mistakes before sending it

There are two main problems with safety behaviors. First, they teach us that *but for the safety behavior, things would have turned out really badly*, thus perpetuating the behaviors and our fears. Second, they can actually impair our performance, as when a capable speaker is overly reliant on notes, which prevents him from engaging with the audience.

In reality, many of our safety behaviors are useless, but we never realize it if we always use them (just like a superstitious practice we're afraid to let go of). We can combine testing our predictions with dropping safety behaviors to directly test whether they're necessary.

BE (MINDFULNESS)

Mindfulness provides several ways to manage our fears, through both the present focus and the acceptance components of the practice. If you haven't read chapter 6 yet, I encourage you to do so before continuing with this section.

Train the breath. Our breath is closely connected to our anxiety: slow and even when we're at ease and fast and sharp when we're afraid. You can feel the contrast right now by first taking a series of fast, deep breaths in and out. Notice how you feel. Then breathe in slowly and out even more slowly. Feel the difference? When we're anxious we often aren't even aware that our breathing is mirroring our anxiety. Once we become more aware of the quality of our breath, we can practice more relaxed breathing:

1 Breathe in gently for a count of two.

2 Exhale slowly to a count of five.

3 Pause after you exhale for a three-count.

4 Repeat from step 1 for 5 to 10 minutes, one to two times per day.

These periods of focused attention on the breath will make it easier to practice relaxed breathing when you need it most. When you feel your anxiety start to increase, practice coming back to the breath.

Focus on the present. Anxiety grabs our attention and pulls it into the future. With practice, we can train the mind to come back to the present. As we disengage from future-oriented fears, we allow anxiety's grip to loosen. Use your senses to bring you into the moment, really paying attention to what you see, feel, and so forth. Keep in mind that there's no need to push away your anxiety, which doesn't work, anyway. Just bring your awareness to your immediate experience, and bring it back when it wanders to your worries.

Direct your attention outward. Certain anxiety states, especially panic, social anxiety, and illness anxiety, lead to a focus on ourselves—our anxiety symptoms, our heart rate, worrisome physical sensations, how we're coming across to the person we're talking to, and so forth. This preoccupation only intensifies our anxiety and discomfort. Mindfulness offers the possibility of training our attention outward, to what's happening in the rest of the world. For example, we can notice what the people around us are doing, what the sky looks like right at this moment, or the shape of a tree we've seen a thousand times but never really noticed. We might find that we not only interrupt our anxiety-fueling self-focus, but we also step into a richer experience of life.

Accept that what you're afraid of could happen. Part of what maintains our fear and worry is mental resistance to what we're afraid might happen. We can't know for certain how things will turn out and yet we keep trying in some way to control the outcome. When we accept that we can't control what happens, we can step out of that tension. We can recognize that our talk could go really badly, we might lose our health, we could be in an accident, and tragedy could befall the people we love. This kind of acceptance is likely to raise anxiety at first—which is probably why we avoid it—and then can lead to a greater sense of peace as we give up the control we never had in the first place.

Embrace uncertainty. In the same vein of acceptance, we can acknowledge—even embrace—the inherent uncertainty in our lives. Who really knows how things will go? That mystery can be terrifying, especially when we'd prefer to control everything all the time. At the same time, it is liberating to align ourselves with the nature of life, which is fluid, surprising, and unpredictable. Since this is the world we inhabit, why not welcome it?

Practicing Exposure Therapy

Wanting to face our fears is one thing; doing it is another. It helps immensely to have a structured approach, which CBT offers in exposure therapy. Effective exposure is:

- **Intentional:** We teach our brains a crucial lesson when we approach our fears *on purpose*, rather than simply not running away when we come into contact with them incidentally.

- **Progressive:** We start with easier things and gradually move up to more challenging ones.

- **Prolonged:** We need to stay with our fears rather than fleeing in order to learn something new.

- **Repetitive:** Multiple confrontations with our fears can disarm them.

With these principles in mind, follow these steps to conquer your fears:

1 **Create a list of ways to face your fears.** Include items on your list that vary in difficulty. Be as creative as you can to come up with a variety of situations that would trigger your fear.

2 **Rate how difficult each one would be.** Make your best guess about how much distress you would feel in each situation; a 0-10 scale tends to work well, but use a different scale if you prefer. See the example that follows.

3 **Arrange your items in descending order of difficulty.** This ordered list of exposure ideas is called your "hierarchy." You might build your hierarchy in a spreadsheet to make it easy to work with. As you review your list, do you notice any big gaps in your numbers, like a jump from a 2 to a 7? If so, look for ways to modify your items to make them easier or harder so you can add intermediate items. For example, doing a difficult activity with a loved one can make it more manageable, and can facilitate a transition to doing it on your own.

Jason was determined to overcome his fear of driving. An abbreviated version of his exposure hierarchy looked like this:

ACTIVITY	DISCOMFORT LEVEL (0–10)
Drive on the expressway alone	9
Drive on the expressway with a friend	7
Drive to work	6
Drive to the grocery store	5
Drive in my neighborhood	4
Sit in driver's seat in parked car	2

4 **Plan and complete your initial exposures.** Choose an item from your hierarchy and schedule a specific time to do it. It's best to choose one of low to moderate difficulty—easy enough that you'll be setting yourself up for success, and hard enough that you'll feel good about having done it.

Be sure to follow the four principles of effective exposure, particularly staying through the discomfort. You don't have to wait until your anxiety is completely gone, but it's good to reach a point at which it's at least beginning to decrease. Running away from an exposure is likely to reinforce our fears. Also take care not to engage in safety behaviors, including compulsions if you're battling OCD.

5 **Continue working up your hierarchy.** Repeat each activity until it starts to feel more manageable. The exposure sessions should be close enough together that the new learning builds on itself; for example, daily practice will be better than weekly. Keep in mind, though, that closer together is not always better, as four exposure sessions on the same day are probably not as effective as four consecutive days of exposure.

As you're ready, move up to more difficult steps. The process will be like climbing a ladder, with success at lower levels enabling continued success as you climb higher. If you're unable to complete a challenging exercise, return to a lower-level one for additional practice before trying the harder one again. It's normal for fear levels to vary between practice sessions, often for no reason we can discern, so don't let temporary setbacks knock you off course. Just keep working your plan.

Refer back to the principles as needed while you do your exposures. You can also incorporate any of the Think Act Be strategies into exposure, such as accepting discomfort. The process of exposure therapy not only will lower your fear but also will increase your willingness and ability to tolerate discomfort.

Chapter Summary and Homework

Fear can direct our lives in many ways if we let it. In this chapter, we reviewed some of the common anxiety conditions and other ways anxiety can color our experience. We also covered many strategies from the Think Act Be framework for reclaiming your life from overwhelming anxiety and fear.

These individual strategies work well together—for example, practicing acceptance of our feared outcome while we do exposure, and testing our predictions for how we expect it to go. By following a systematic program for exposure, we can transform our determination to conquer our fears into real progress.

When you're ready to face your fears, here are ways to get started:

1 Complete a CBT diagram of your fears, identifying your relevant thoughts, feelings, and behaviors and their relationships.

2 Look for subtle ways that fear affects you that aren't immediately apparent.

3 Choose strategies from the Think, Act, and Be categories to practice in the coming days.

4 If you have specific fears that lend themselves well to exposure therapy, begin with step 1 and work consistently through the plan.

5 Balance the tough work of facing your fear with consistent self-care (see chapter 10). Being good to yourself will help you through this process.

CHAPTER NINE

Keep Calm: Manage Excessive Anger

Anger can be a powerful emotional experience, for better or worse. In this chapter, we'll examine problematic anger and ways of managing it effectively.

Alan was taken aback when he caught a glimpse of himself in the mirror as he waited on hold. The flushed face and furious expression it wore almost made him laugh. "I look like a maniac," he thought to himself. His ordeal had started 45 minutes earlier when he called to exchange a product he had ordered. It took him several tries to get through the automated prompts, as the system kept placing him on hold and then disconnecting after several minutes. By the time he reached a human being he was starting to see red.

The voice on the other end didn't seem very sympathetic when he complained about the difficulty getting through, and when he explained his request for an exchange, she recited the company policy: "There is a 14-day window for returns or exchanges, and unfortunately there are no exceptions." Alan gritted his teeth and described his extenuating circumstances: Not receiving the order till after the 14 days had passed, his recent move, the address update that hadn't registered. . . . The representative replied with irritating calmness, "Sir, it is the customer's responsibility to update their address of record."

Furious, Alan replied, "I'd like to speak with someone who isn't hard of hearing."

"One moment while I transfer you." After five minutes of music, the line went dead. It was all Alan could do not to throw his phone against the wall. Twenty minutes later, he had a similar conversation and unleashed a string of expletives, ending by asking to "speak to someone who actually gives a damn about customer service."

We've all experienced irritating situations, whether they're with customer service representatives, customers, friends, spouses, parents, kids, bosses, or strangers. When channeled appropriately, anger can be a force for good. However, excessive anger has unhealthy effects, both on our health and our relationships.

Let's begin by exploring what anger is and how it's expressed, and then we'll turn to ways of managing it.

Understanding Anger

There are many words to describe our experiences of anger. Annoyance and irritation describe some milder forms of anger, whereas rage and fury suggest more intense emotional states. The quality of our anger will vary, as well. We'll feel *frustrated* when our aims are thwarted, *exasperated* when our anger mixes with disbelief, *outraged* when we perceive a gross violation of what's right. Other descriptions of anger have their own nuances: *resentful, bitter, indignant, livid, apoplectic, incensed, vexed, cross, seething, irate*, and so forth.

What do all of these descriptions have in common? In one way or another there is the sense of *having been wronged*. We have expectations of how we want things to go and when someone or something causes a worse outcome than we expected, we're liable to get angry.

The thoughts we have when things don't go our way are central to the degree of anger we feel. During Alan's customer service experience, he had thought to himself, "This is a complete waste of my time." Just below his conscious awareness was the related thought, "These people don't care that they're wasting my time." That interpretation is what sent him over the edge into feelings of rage.

Alan also had thoughts related to expressing his anger. As his anger built, he began to feel like he needed to punish the person he was talking to for mistreating him. "They need to know I'm not a sucker who can be pushed around," he told himself.

Unbeknownst to Alan, his body was having its own set of reactions. His blood pressure and heart rate had increased as attention had narrowed in on the target of his anger. His breathing also had quickened as he entered a full activation of his sympathetic nervous system, more fight than flight. He was ready for battle.

We can break down the components of anger to better understand it and to find places in the process to intervene. Our model of anger begins with a triggering situation—some violation of our expectation of how we should be treated. Our resulting thoughts, driven by our core beliefs (see chapter 5), will lead to emotional and physical reactions. Together these thoughts, feelings, and physical sensations comprise our subjective experience of anger.

We make an important distinction in this model between our *experience* of anger and our *expression* of anger. The former clearly influences the latter, of course, since we have to experience anger before expressing it. However, we can exercise some choice in whether and how we act on our anger.

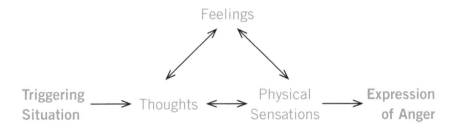

Experience of Anger

For example, when someone cuts us off in traffic we might decide to let our grievance go rather than retaliating. Or we might channel our anger into a measured response, taking care to keep our wits about us. At other times, we might give full vent to our wrath, attacking the target of our anger with harsh words or even physical actions. At the extreme the outcome of uncontrolled anger can include abuse or even homicide.

Our thoughts will strongly influence how we express our anger. We're more likely to act on our anger when we have beliefs like *if people treat me badly, I need to punish them.* These kinds of beliefs give rise to permission-giving thoughts that facilitate our anger expression—thoughts like, "I should teach them a lesson," or "They deserve it."

The Utility of Anger

As with our other emotions, anger exists for good reason. Anger is a highly energized state and can give us the impetus to stand up for ourselves and for what is right. For example, cars in my neighborhood kept running red lights at the intersection where families cross a busy road to get to the playground, including several times as we waited to cross with our own kids. My sense of what was right—kids need a safe intersection to get across the street—had been violated, and my resulting anger led me to contact our local commissioner about having more safety measures added to the intersection. Anger can be extremely motivating.

Anger is also a clear sign to others that they have violated our boundaries. We generally pay attention when someone is mad, so anger can actually facilitate clear communication. Indeed, under-expressing anger can be as much of a problem as overexpressing it. Just as we saw with anxiety, anger becomes a problem when we experience it to such a degree that its costs outweigh its bene-fits. We might feel angry all the time, even for no apparent reason. We may be quick to make faulty interpretations that lead to anger, like assuming people are criticizing us when in fact they are not. Maybe we have a hard time coming down from episodes of anger, or we express anger in unhealthy ways.

Several psychological conditions can lead to problems with anger. Although depression is linked most obviously to feeling down, irri-tability is a very common symptom. Irritability or even aggression can also be part of the hyperarousal in PTSD. The pervasive worry in GAD often leads to irritability, as well. Similarly, individuals with OCD may get angry if they see others as triggering their obses-sions or thwarting their compulsions. It is important to treat an underlying condition that may be contributing to excessive anger. As the condition improves, anger and irritability should diminish.

What Contributes to Excessive Anger?

People vary in how often and how intensely they experience and express anger. The following mental processes have been linked to high anger levels.

SELECTIVE ATTENTION

People prone to anger tend to pay attention to things that trigger anger. A person might be primed to notice other drivers' offensive behaviors, for example, or to focus on things his or her partner says that might be critical. The more we look for these things, the more cause we'll find to be angry.

BIASED THINKING

As we saw in chapter 5, our core beliefs drive our thoughts in triggering situations. The more we interpret others' actions as hostile, inconsiderate, and so forth, the more we'll experience anger.

RUMINATION

It's easy to get stuck in our heads about things that made us angry, turning them over and over. We'll replay interactions that upset us, wonder how others could treat us so unfairly, and even create scripts for irritating arguments that may never happen. Dwelling on anger-related memories and moods only exacerbates our anger.

Strategies for Dealing with Excessive Anger

Anger typically is fast and impulsive. We describe an angry person as being quick-tempered or a hothead. We feel a flash of anger and are tempted to lash out. We need ways to slow down, cool things off, and find space to choose how we react.

Each of the strategies for defusing anger is a way to keep you in the driver's seat, rather than being hijacked by emotion. The techniques presented here will fall into the familiar categories of Think (cognitive), Act (behavioral), and Be (mindfulness).

THINK (COGNITIVE)

- **Know your triggers.** Most of us have people or situations that consistently test our patience. Common examples include driving, being pressed for time, or certain topics of disagreement with a loved one. Many of the strategies for dealing with anger require knowing in advance what's likely to irritate us. Take some time to write down your common triggers.

- **Remember the costs of excessive anger.** When you are angry, it's easy to ignore the consequences of indulging in it. What has anger cost you that motivates you to work on managing it? How has it affected your peace of mind? Your closest relationships? Your professional life?

- **Examine your thoughts.** Use the techniques from chapter 4 to identify and examine your anger-related thoughts. Look for thinking errors that may be fueling your anger. Are there alternative beliefs or explanations that would make more sense and be less irritating?

PLANNING IN ADVANCE
TO MANAGE ANGER

Angry episodes don't just happen—they generally have specific antecedents. We can often understand in hindsight the chain of events that led to our anger. These conditions were like dry wood and all it took was a spark to ignite a blaze of anger. With practice, we can start to look down the road and see warning signs before we fly off the handle. Once we see what's ahead we can use the strategies that work well for us: adopting a helpful mind-set, lowering our emotional arousal with a few calming breaths, allowing ourselves adequate time to minimize a sense of pressure, and other techniques presented in this chapter. We can't always avoid episodes of anger, but we can prevent perfect setups by planning in advance when possible.

The basement lights were on again. Rick swore aloud. "The kids never remember to turn off the lights," he thought with irritation. Then he realized—it was only the second time this week. Rick still wanted his kids to be more consistent, but he felt less annoyed after checking his thinking.

It can be unrealistic to change our thinking in the heat of the moment, as anger may overpower our reason. At those times simply note the thoughts that are going through your head and return to evaluate them when you're feeling calmer.

- **Question your "shoulds."** One word that often shows up in our anger-inducing thoughts is "should":

  > "This shouldn't be so hard."

  > "They should treat me better."

  > "These drivers should go faster."

  These "shoulds" generally reflect an error in thinking, for while we might *prefer* a certain outcome, there's no actual rule that's being violated. Checking our sense of violation can diminish unnecessary anger.

- **Talk yourself down.** Practice talking to yourself the way you would to a friend who's upset. Come up with words or phrases that encourage you to calm down when you're starting to wind up. Examples include:

  > "Take it easy."

  > "Be cool."

  > "Breathe through this."

  > "No need to get bent out of shape."

- **Notice when you're feeding anger-related thoughts.** We can fuel our own anger even without any ongoing stimulus by mentally going over things that upset us. Ruminating on our anger in this way can include imagined conversations that we find upsetting—even getting mad about made-up interactions! Mindfulness practices are well suited to help redirect rumination (see chapter 6).

- **Remember your larger goal.** Anger narrows our focus onto the target of our anger, which can crowd out our bigger goals. For example, we might lose sight of the relationship we're trying to foster with our kids when we're frustrated with them. Write down the ways in which anger has interfered with your goals. When you feel anger rising, remind yourself of the things that are important to you.

- **Question your explanations of others' behavior.** When we make a mistake, we tend to find causes outside of ourselves to account for them. When others make mistakes, we blame them on the person. For example, I used to get annoyed with drivers who had their lights off at night and didn't turn them on when I toggled my high beams; I assumed they must be morons. Then one night I did it myself, getting all the way to my destination without realizing I'd forgotten to turn on my lights. I realized we can all make this mistake, and I stopped getting annoyed with these drivers.

  When you notice that you're attributing others' faults to their character, ask yourself if there's a kinder and more accurate explanation. Maybe the driver who cut you off is on the phone with the doctor about his sick child, rather than simply being "a jerk." The attributions we make for others' behavior have a big impact on our anger.

- **Question your "have to" assumptions.** Anger can lead to imperatives: "I have to teach that driver a lesson," "My child has to stop talking back to me," "You have to admit I'm right." These thoughts can compel us to take actions we'll soon regret because with few exceptions, the thoughts are overstated preferences. For example, I might *really want* you to admit I'm right—and if you don't, life will go on. Mindful acceptance (see chapter 6) is a good fit here.

- **Question the utility of angry responses.** Anger is good at justifying itself, both its presence and the actions it can lead to. For example, most drivers who retaliate against other drivers say they do so to teach the drivers a lesson so they'll improve their driving. Does it help? We don't have data to answer that question directly, but consider this: Have you ever resolved to be a better driver because of an angry motorist's behavior toward you? With that idea in mind, beware of thoughts that make lashing out in anger sound like a good plan.

ACT (BEHAVIORAL)

Our experience and expression of anger also depend on the behaviors we practice. Consider the following actions that can help you manage your anger.

Get enough sleep. As my colleagues at the University of Pennsylvania have shown, being sleep deprived lowers our ability to tolerate minor frustrations. Inadequate sleep can also lower our inhibitions, increasing our risk for aggression and even violence. See chapter 10 for more on sleep.

Notice other states of physical discomfort. Our physical state has a big influence on our irritability and anger. When we're hungry, in pain, or otherwise uncomfortable, we're going to have a harder time controlling our anger. Personally I've had countless times when I've gotten cranky while cooking dinner, not realizing I was overheating. Something as simple as taking off my sweater can work wonders. The more we tend to our physical well-being, the less prone we'll be to problematic anger.

Provide yourself with adequate time. When we're running late we tend to feel stressed out and impatient—a perfect recipe for an angry outburst if things don't go our way. Give yourself enough time for what you need to do to prevent unnecessary stress and anger.

Postpone arguments when necessary. Most disagreements don't have to be resolved immediately. If you find that conflict is escalating or you're reaching your boiling point, plan to pause the discussion until you've calmed down. Our anger can tell us we need to resolve this *now*, but ask yourself—have you ever regretted dealing with something calmly versus in the heat of anger?

Assert your needs. Many of us alternate between passivity and aggression when others do things that interfere with our needs. When we swallow our anger, we create pressure that eventually can come out all at once.

> Martin lay in bed listening to his neighbor's loud music—it was the fourth night this week he'd been kept awake by it. Finally he'd had enough. Throwing on his robe and slippers, he walked to his neighbor's apartment and pounded on the door. When his neighbor finally opened it, Martin started screaming at him.

We can deal with violations of our needs more effectively when we address them as they happen versus storing them up and accumulating frustration and resentment. See the Resources section to learn more about assertiveness.

BE (MINDFULNESS)

The tools of mindfulness can be invaluable when emotions are hot and it's hard to think. Anger compels us to act impulsively; as Dr. Aaron T. Beck has suggested, we can reframe anger as signaling an imperative *not* to act, since we'll probably regret actions we take in anger even though our thoughts in the heat of the moment will tell us otherwise. Often the best thing to do when we're angry is nothing. I've included in this section some relaxation techniques, which are not mindfulness practices in the strictest sense but have considerable overlap with a mindfulness approach.

- **Focus on the present to disengage from anger rumination.** As discussed earlier, ruminating on things that upset us only perpetuates our anger, yet it isn't easy to disengage from these repetitive thoughts. We can use whatever we're doing as a focal point to connect our attention to the present, rather than staying in our heads. For example, if we're making dinner, we can tune in to the sensations of chopping vegetables, the sounds of sautéing, the smells of onion and garlic cooking, and so forth. See chapter 6 for more on mindfulness in daily activities.

- **Practice acceptance.** So much of our anger stems from the belief that things *should* be different than they are. Through mindful awareness we let go of these judgments. Rather than railing against outcomes we don't like, we can open to what is happening. This practice can be particularly helpful for releasing resentful rumination.

- **Recognize your anger.** Through the practice of mindfulness, we can become more aware of our anger-related thoughts, feelings, and behaviors. For example, we might notice that we're feeling tense and ready for a fight as we broach a difficult topic with our spouse. This awareness gives us opportunities for managing our anger before it leads us to do things we regret.

- **Learn your patterns.** Mindfulness can also raise our awareness of certain times or situations when we tend toward anger.

Gene realized he fell easily into irritability and impatience most nights after dinner. He would be short with his family members and quick to get frustrated. By stepping out of autopilot mode, he was able to use strategies for managing his emotions at these vulnerable times.

- **Identify your primary emotions.** Anger often comes from other emotions. For example, we might feel hurt or rejected and respond with anger, which in a way might be a more comfortable emotion for us. Or perhaps we feel fear that triggers us to lash out, as when a fellow driver nearly causes an accident and our fear response quickly morphs into rage. Notice what might be beneath your anger at times. Once we're aware of a feeling that led to anger, we can deal with the source of the emotion rather than getting lost in the overlay of anger.

- **Relax.** Anger is a state of tension, and physical relaxation can defuse it. A simple reminder to ourselves to relax, accompanied by a calming breath, can lessen our tension. It also helps to practice deep relaxation when we're not in the grip of anger so that we can let go of tension on command (see section on progressive muscle relaxation on pages 170–171).

- **Breathe with your anger.** We don't have to react to our anger, but instead can learn to tolerate it. By breathing with the anger, we can open to the experience of being angry, allowing it to run its course like a wave that rises, crests, and falls. Mindful breathing will also engage your parasympathetic nervous system, which quiets the fight-or-flight response.

- **Observe the anger.** We can take a small step back from our anger by taking the role of observer of our experiences. Rather than identifying 100 percent with being angry, we can maintain some perspective on our reactions, seeing them as passing through us. When we watch our angry reactions like this we start to recognize that we don't have to act on the thoughts and feelings.

MEDITATION FOR MANAGING ANGER

In the following practice we use the body and the breath as vehicles to manage unresolved anger.

1. Begin with a few moments of basic breath meditation (see page 95). Feel your body and any sensations that are present from your toes to your head.

2. Picture as vividly as possible the circumstances that led to your anger, opening to the emotions they provoke.

3. Notice where the anger expresses itself in the body— for example, a clenched jaw or a knot in the stomach. Breathe with these physical manifestations of anger. Bring compassion to your experience, making room for the emo- tion. Let it be what it is. Take care not to resist the feel- ings or criticize yourself for the reactions you're having.

4. Practice being the witness of your own experience, observ- ing your emotions without becoming completely entangled in them. If you struggle to take the role of observer, that's OK, too—it's easy to get wrapped up in anger. If at any point you feel overwhelmed with emotion, gently direct the attention to the breath until the grip of anger loosens.

5. Continue to breathe with the physical sensations for as long as you like, noticing how emotions change over time. When the intensity of the anger has abated, bring the attention back to the breath before opening your eyes. Notice how you feel.

This meditation allows us to practice pausing between feeling angry and reacting, giving us greater choice in how we manage strong emotions.

Chapter Summary and Homework

Uncontrolled anger can lead to conflict, aggression, and even violence. In this chapter, we examined the factors that lead to excessive anger and described ways to manage it. Keep in mind that the goal is not to banish anger from our lives. Instead, we can learn to keep it in check. Things to practice from this chapter include:

1 Complete a diagram for a specific situation that made you angry to learn more about your own experience of anger.

2 Use a thought record to capture and examine some of your anger-related thoughts for a situation that comes up.

3 Begin to note situations in which you'd like to practice managing your anger.

4 Choose one or two techniques from the Think, Act, and Be categories to start practicing.

5 Write down how each technique works for you, and add new ones as needed.

6 Refer to your list of strategies often to remind yourself of the best ways for you to manage your anger.

CHAPTER TEN

Be Kind to Yourself

Up to this point, we've covered the fundamentals of cognitive, behavioral, and mindfulness-based strategies, and we've seen how these practices can help us manage strong emotions. In this chapter, we examine practical ways of taking care of ourselves—mind, body, and spirit.

John grimaced as the alarm clock went off. "You have to start getting to bed earlier," he told himself as he sat up and rubbed his eyes.

After taking a quick shower, John grabbed a cup of coffee and a frozen waffle, eating fast as he thought about the big day ahead at work. As he put his dishes in the sink, he braced himself to face the morning rush hour.

In the car he divided his attention between listening to the radio news with its daily reminder of all that was wrong in the world and worrying about all the ways he could mess up at work today.

The morning went surprisingly well and by noon John was famished and ready for a break; however, when his coworkers invited him to join them for lunch at the deli, John decided he hadn't gotten enough done to take a real lunch break. Instead he grabbed some snacks from the vending machine to eat at his desk, along with a soda for the caffeine and sugar boost.

He made three more trips to the vending machine that afternoon for more peanut butter crackers and M&Ms—once because he was hungry, once when he was bored and anxious, and once in the late afternoon for another diet cola to power him through his 4 o'clock slump.

After the second stressful commute of the day, John thought about hitting the gym before dinner, but wasn't sure he had the energy. Instead he took the leftover pizza and two beers out of the refrigerator and ate in front of the TV. Afterward he finished a pint of ice cream.

Around midnight John started to nod off in front of the TV. His sleep hadn't been good lately so he tried his best not to wake himself up as he walked upstairs to bed. Despite his desperate wishes to the contrary, he was fully awake as soon as his head hit the pillow. "I'm going to be a wreck tomorrow," he thought as he tried harder to fall asleep.

After tossing and turning for an hour, John turned the TV back on to help him sleep. It was still on the next morning when his alarm went off, and John cringed when he realized it was only Tuesday. "You've got to stop doing this to yourself," he said.

John is stuck in a cycle of behaviors that are depleting his energy and hurting his mood. As the figure below demonstrates, his habits affect his mood and his energy, which in turn perpetuate his habits.

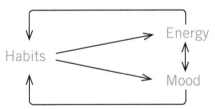

For example, John's caffeine consumption interferes with his sleep, which makes him tired and unmotivated to exercise. The lack of exercise doesn't help his mood or his energy levels, which compels him to continue relying on caffeine for energy in the daytime and on alcohol to unwind and fall asleep at night. On top of these unhelpful habits, John consistently second-guesses and criticizes himself.

What would we think if John had a life coach who was directing him to act in these ways? We would probably think he had a terrible coach, guiding him to continue these bad habits. We might even wonder if the coach really cared about John. And yet the reality is that in a very real way, John was acting as his own coach and was giving himself the instructions he was following.

Let's consider some of the most important ways to take care of ourselves that help us feel good and move toward our goals.

Sleep Tight

We need adequate sleep to function at our best. Unfortunately, millions of adults in the United States are sleep deprived, either because they don't give themselves enough time in bed or because they have insomnia.

HOW MUCH SLEEP DO YOU NEED?

Most of us have heard that we need eight hours of sleep per night. In reality, it's not quite that simple. The latest guidelines from the National Sleep Foundation recommend seven to nine hours of sleep per night for most adults (seven to eight for older adults). A minority of individuals actually need only six hours.

How do you figure out where you fall in that range? Consider tracking your sleep for two weeks, noting the time you went to bed and the time you got out of bed. Subtract the approximate amount of time you were awake at the beginning, middle, and end of the night. Based on the numbers for each night, you can calculate the average amount of sleep you're getting.

For example, let's say you go to bed at 10:30 p.m. and get up at 6:30 a.m., so you're in bed for eight hours. It takes you 10 minutes to fall asleep and you're generally awake in the night for 20 minutes or so, and then sleep through until your alarm at 6:30 a.m. Your total sleep time for this night would be eight hours minus 30 minutes, so seven and a half hours of sleep.

If you often feel sleepy during the day and you don't suffer from a medical condition that would account for it (e.g., sleep apnea), you probably need more sleep than you're getting. If you wake up consistently feeling relatively refreshed and aren't overly sleepy during the day (and aren't relying on caffeine or other stimulants to stay awake), you're probably getting enough sleep.

PROBLEMS FROM TOO LITTLE SLEEP

Virtually every area of our life suffers when we're not getting enough sleep: our mood, energy, concentration, relationships, work performance, driving ability, and more. Nevertheless, countless men and women push through the sleepiness, use stimulants to keep going, and ignore the likely costs of missed sleep. It can be hard to make sleep a priority when it seems like wasted time and that we're doing nothing. Hanging out with friends, getting more work done, watching our favorite shows, and countless other activities compete with our need for sleep.

However, sleep is anything but a state of inactivity. While our bodies might be still, our brains are busy at work, as getting the proper amount of sleep leads to better learning and memory. Sleep also facilitates healing in our bodies, and sleep deprivation has been shown to raise levels of inflammatory markers in the body. When we deprive ourselves of sleep, it is to our own detriment.

If you want to get more sleep but have struggled to make it a priority, consider what you might tell a good friend. How might you help that friend using the tools of CBT? Like any other task, we would plan a specific time to get in bed, depending on when we planned to get up and how much sleep we were aiming for. We might also set an alarm to alert us when we should start our bedtime routine. Refer to chapter 7, as many of the practices presented there apply to the problem of delaying our bedtime.

As you start to feel the reward from getting more sleep, you'll be motivated to continue prioritizing your rest. You might also find you're sharper and more productive during the day, which can make up for having fewer hours of awake time.

HOW TO FIX A BROKEN SLEEP CYCLE

But what if your problem isn't getting in bed on time—what if you're spending plenty of time in bed and yet aren't able to sleep? If you consistently struggle to fall asleep or stay asleep, or if you wake up long before you intend to, you may be suffering from insomnia along with millions of other U.S. adults. Insomnia often starts with a clearly caused sleep disruption. We may be taking a medication that interferes with our sleep or perhaps work stress is keeping us up at night.

Understandably we'll try to make up for the sleep we're losing by going to bed earlier, sleeping in after a bad night's sleep, or taking naps. Unfortunately, we often end up making it worse in the process. If you sleep in, for example, you're probably going to have a hard time falling asleep that night. Lying in bed unable to sleep usually leads to anxiety about sleep, which aggravates the insomnia. As a result, we may continue to sleep poorly even after the original issue (e.g., work stress) has been resolved.

The number one treatment for chronic difficulty sleeping is cognitive behavioral therapy for insomnia (CBT-I). The guidelines from CBT-I are good sleep practices in general, and include:

- Going to bed and getting up at the same time every day

- Planning to be in bed only for the amount of time you're actually able to sleep

- Using the bed for sleeping only (sex is an exception) to strengthen the "bed equals sleep" association

- Getting out of bed if you're having a hard time sleeping to break the link between bed and being anxious about not sleeping

- Challenging unhelpful thoughts about sleep (e.g., catastrophizing about how terrible the next day will be due to bad sleep)

- Practicing relaxation to counteract the tension and anxiety that typically go along with insomnia

- Practicing mindful awareness and acceptance to interrupt sleep-related worries and to let go of efforts to force yourself asleep

- Following other practices that promote good sleep, like limiting caffeine intake (especially after lunchtime); making the bedroom cool, dark, and quiet; keeping electronics out of the bedroom; and exercising regularly

- Avoiding napping in general, which can make it harder to sleep well at night

- Having a winding-down routine that signals your body and brain that bedtime is approaching (e.g., gently stretching, reading for pleasure, or drinking a cup of herbal tea)

If you've been struggling with poor sleep, are there sleep guidelines you'd like to follow this week? Write your plans in your notebook.

Nourish Your Body and Brain

It's well known that foods we put in our bodies affect our physical health. For example, if we eat large amounts of sugar, we'll be more prone to obesity and related health problems like type 2 diabetes. We'll also experience spikes in our blood sugar followed by crashes, leading to low energy and sugar cravings that continue the cycle.

There is mounting evidence that our diet also has a big impact on our mental and emotional well-being, which has led to a new mental health field called nutritional psychiatry/psychology.

EATING FOR MENTAL HEALTH

While specific dietary recommendations for mental health vary, they consistently call for eating minimally processed food—in particular, lots of vegetables and fruits, nuts, legumes, potatoes, whole grains, fish, and healthy fats like olive oil. Foods to limit or avoid include highly processed foods, refined sugar, fast food, and trans fats (e.g., hydrogenated oil).

These recommendations are similar to the "Mediterranean diet" and are based on studies over the past decade showing that these dietary habits significantly affect mental health. For example, a 2009 study in the *British Journal of Psychiatry* found that a diet high in processed food raised the odds of developing depression by as much as 58 percent over a five-year period. Other research has shown similar effects of diet on anxiety disorders.

Based on these associations, the first study of its kind used a Mediterranean-style diet plus fish oil supplements as a treatment for depression. Results showed that the dietary changes led to greater improvement than did the control condition, producing an average reduction in depression symptoms of nearly 50 percent by three months, which was maintained at six months.

One of the advantages of the Mediterranean diet, besides the health benefits, is that it also tends to be appealing since it's not overly restrictive. The guidelines allow for a wide variety of colorful fruits and vegetables, plenty of satisfying healthy fats, and sufficient protein.

Researchers have tried to determine how diet affects our mental health, and a key factor seems to be inflammation. For example, one study found that a diet high in foods that trigger the body's inflammation response more than doubled a person's odds for developing depression. Interestingly, this association may hold only for women, though men would do well to follow the same dietary guidelines.

"The more one eats a diet rich in fruits and vegetables, high in healthy fats, nuts, and fish, and low in processed food (a Mediterranean-style diet), the more one is protected from developing a mental disorder." —Julia J. Rucklidge and Bonnie J. Kaplan

CHALLENGES TO EATING FOR HEALTH

Given the considerable advantages of eating a healthy diet, what makes it so hard for so many people to follow these guidelines? Much of the problem is simply the inconvenience. Consider John from earlier in this chapter. When he was pressed for time, it was easy to reach for convenience foods like frozen waffles and vending-machine snacks. When you're hurrying through the train station and need to grab something on the go, there are countless quick, easy, and less healthy options. The same is true at home: Eating well requires advance planning, like picking recipes, making a grocery list, going to the grocery store, and learning how to cook if we don't already know how. In contrast, highly processed options are often as easy as opening a bag.

Convenience foods also tend to provide a triple hit of fat, sugar, and salt, which is a highly reinforcing combination. We face an uphill struggle if we intend to eat for health, and can end up consuming foods that are mostly various shades of tan, made from ingredients we don't recognize and can't pronounce. If you're committed to eating better, make a plan for moving toward that goal. I've included a link to information from the Mayo Clinic in the Resources section to get you started. Based on the benefits of a healthy diet—including not just our mental health but also better physical health and a longer life—the investment in ourselves is well worth the effort.

Move Your Body

As with a sound diet, consistent exercise is an essential part of all aspects of health. The benefits of exercise on physical health are no secret; research studies have shown that exercise also has positive effects on psychological conditions like anxiety, depression, eating disorders, and substance use disorders, as well as chronic pain and neurodegenerative conditions like Alzheimer's disease. The effects of exercise have been studied most with depression, for which the benefits tend to be quite large. Both aerobic (e.g., running) and anaerobic (e.g., weight lifting) exercise can improve mental health.

HOW DOES EXERCISE HELP?

There are many avenues whereby exercise can be beneficial. These include:

- Better sleep, which is associated with improved mental health

- A release of endorphins, the body's natural "feel good" chemicals

- A sense of accomplishment from having exercised and from increased fitness

- Distraction from unhealthy thought patterns like rumination

- Increased blood flow to the brain

- Improvement in executive functions like organization and focus

- Social contact with others who are exercising

- Spending time outdoors (when applicable); see the section "Spend Time Outside" (page 174) on being in nature

HOW TO GET STARTED

If you're ready to take advantage of the many benefits of exercise, follow the steps from chapter 3 for behavioral activation:

1 Start by defining what's important to you about physical activity. For example, is it about doing something that brings you joy or feeling like you're taking care of yourself?

2 Find activities you enjoy, which may not even fall under the label "exercise." They might include going for walks with a friend, playing tennis, or taking a dance class, for example. The more you enjoy the movement, the more motivated you'll be to do it consistently.

3 Plan specific times to exercise, and schedule them in your calendar. Start gradually so you won't feel overwhelmed by your goals.

With thoughtful planning, you can add regular exercise into your routine and enjoy the all-around positive effects on your well-being.

Manage Stress

Anything that creates a demand on our physical, mental, or emotional resources will produce some amount of stress, making stress an unavoidable part of life. Just like with our emotions, the goal is not to eliminate stress from our lives but to learn how to manage it effectively. In his seminal work, Hungarian endocrinologist Hans Selye revealed there is a common stress response regardless of the source of the stress. It doesn't matter whether we're being chased by an alligator or giving a speech—the sympathetic nervous system will engage to help us meet the challenge.

"On an incredibly simplistic level, you can think of depression as occurring when your cortex thinks an abstract negative thought and manages to convince the rest of the brain that this is as real as a physical stressor." —Robert Sapolsky, Why Zebras Don't Get Ulcers

Selye discovered we handle short-term stress really well: Our body mounts a response, we deal with the situation, and our parasympathetic nervous system eases us back down to our baseline. However, when the stress goes on and on, our body and brain become worn down.

The cumulative effects of long-term stress include impaired function of the immune system, digestive and cardiac problems, and psychological illness. In addition to the long-term effects of chronic stress, it's simply not enjoyable to live in a constant state of high alert.

The first step in managing stress is awareness. Start simply by becoming curious about how you respond to stress, allowing the mind to open to what you're experiencing. For example:

- Are you clenching your jaw?

- Is your stomach tight?

- Are you holding tension in your neck and shoulders?

- What is the quality of your breath like?

- What are your thoughts up to?

With practice, we can sharpen our recognition of what stress feels like in our bodies and minds, so that we can begin to let it go. Practicing mindfulness (see chapter 6) can help in this regard.

Effective ways of managing the stress in our lives include:

- Minimizing unnecessary stress (e.g., steering clear of people who create stress)

- Saying "no" to commitments when we're already overextended

- Relaxing rigid and unrealistic standards for ourselves (e.g., I *have* to finish this project today)

- Focusing on what's happening right in the present

- Taking slow breaths

- Practicing meditation

- Taking a yoga class

- Getting regular exercise

- Doing progressive muscle relaxation (see pages 170–171)

- Taking short breaks throughout the day

- Going on vacation

- Protecting time away from work each day and on the weekend

- Challenging unhelpful thoughts about what you *should* be doing

- Carving out time for yourself to do relaxing activities you enjoy like reading or taking a warm bath

Progressive Muscle Relaxation

Follow these steps to reach a deep state of relaxation.

1 Find a quiet place where you won't be disturbed. Silence your phone.

2 Sit in a chair with your legs stretched out in front of you, heels on the floor. Make any necessary adjustments to get comfortable. Allow your eyes to close.

3 Alternately tense and then relax the major muscle groups in your body, starting with your feet and working your way up. Create a moderate degree of muscular tension in each area of the body for a few seconds. Then release the tension all at once, really noticing the contrast as you move from tense to relaxed. Continue to relax for 30 to 60 seconds before tensing the next group of muscles.

The sequence can include:

Lower legs: One leg at a time, pull your toes toward you to create tension along your shin.

Thighs: One leg at a time, flex your leg, tensing the quadriceps muscle in the front of your thigh.

Glutes: Squeeze your buttock muscles.

Abdomen: Tense your stomach muscles and pull your navel in toward your spine.

Breath: Take a deep breath in, allowing it to expand your chest, and hold it. Release tension when you exhale.

Upper arms: One arm at a time, tense the muscles in each upper arm.

Forearms and hands: One arm at a time, make a fist and pull your hand backward toward your elbow, creating tension through your hand, wrist, and forearm.

Neck and upper back: Shrug your shoulders up toward your ears.

Face and scalp: Raise your eyebrows while simultaneously scrunching your eyes tightly closed (you may need to remove contact lenses for this one).

4 Take a few nice, slow breaths as you release any remaining muscle tension, letting your entire body enter a state of deep relaxation.

5 Bring your attention to your breath. Follow the sensations of breathing in and out. With each exhalation, mentally say to yourself a single word that you associate with relaxation (e.g., "peace," "calm," "breathe," etc.). Continue saying this word in your mind each time you exhale, for three to five minutes.

6 Slowly return your awareness to where you are. Begin to wiggle your toes and fingers. When you're ready, open your eyes. Notice how you feel.

7 Practice this sequence at least once per day (ideally twice).

8 Over time you can abbreviate the practice as you get more adept at letting go of tension. You can do both legs or both arms at once, for example, and only do the muscle groups where you tend to hold tension.

By pairing deep relaxation with a word and an exhale, you'll be training your mind and body to enter a state of relaxation on cue. When you find yourself starting to feel tense and stressed, you can take a calming breath, say your word as you exhale, and feel the benefits of all your progressive muscle relaxation training.

In a world that puts a premium on constant busyness, it can feel like we can't afford to take time to relax. However, this time is never wasted and should not be considered a luxury. By investing in your own well-being, you'll be more productive and more enjoyable to be around.

Engage with the Real World

In the last decade, technology has permeated all areas of our lives. You may remember a time, like I do, when there were no smartphones or even cell phones, no laptop computers, no social media or e-mail. The advent of these technologies has brought many benefits, like rapid sharing of ideas and the ability to connect quickly and effortlessly with people around the globe.

At the same time, there are potential downsides to the ubiquity of technology. Many research studies have begun to examine the effects of various technologies on our well-being. Their findings include:

- People who use Facebook more end up less happy over time, and less satisfied with their lives.

- Seeing others as happier or more successful in their social media posts leads people to experience decreases in self-esteem and increases in anxiety and jealousy.

- Greater smartphone use at home is associated with greater work–home conflict.

- More time spent on technology is linked with greater burnout.

- A greater presence of technology in the bedroom is associated with worse sleep.

Technology can be highly addicting, so it's easy to fall into patterns of overuse. If you've been with a loved one who is constantly on their phone, you know firsthand the potential toll that technological intrusions can take on relationships. And yet, even as we find others' constant use irritating, we may engage in the same behaviors ourselves.

Take a few moments to think about your own relationship with your phone and other screens, and notice over the next few days how often you're turning to your phone or tablet. While a whole world might await us on our smartphones, in another sense the scene never changes if we're glued to a screen. Consider whether it may be a good idea to increase the time you spend immersed in real life—for example:

- Turn on your "Do Not Disturb" function when you want a break from your phone.

- Leave your phone at home sometimes.

- Turn off notifications so your phone isn't prompting you to interact with it.

- Make mealtime a technology-free zone.

- Make social media less easily available (e.g., uninstall it from your smartphone).

- Minimize the number of apps you use, since each one increases the reasons you'll find to be on your phone.

- Trade your smartphone for a traditional cell phone. While I know this option sounds extreme, I found it liberating when I did it for three years.

Spend Time Outside

Being outdoors is good for our well-being. For example, living in "greener" neighborhoods is associated with better mental health. A study by Ian Alcock and his collaborators found that those who moved to a greener area had a subsequent improvement in their mental health that was maintained through a three-year follow-up period. Part of the beneficial effect of greener neighborhoods seems to come from the greater ability to walk for recreation; green areas like parks also serve as a meeting place for neighborhood friends, facilitating social connection.

There also appears to be a direct benefit of being in natural environments that weren't constructed by humans; for example, we can enjoy the natural beauty of our surroundings while hiking in the woods, perhaps even finding a sense of spiritual connection. Time in nature also gives us a break from dealing with traffic, constant bombardment by advertising and entertainment, and automatic vigilance for potentially threatening people.

"Those who contemplate the beauty of the earth find reserves of strength that will endure as long as life lasts. There is something infinitely healing in the repeated refrains of nature—the assurance that dawn comes after night, and spring after winter."
—Rachel Carson

There is also evidence from laboratory studies that viewing nature scenes engages the parasympathetic nervous system, helping a person recover after encountering a stressor. Related findings showed that going for a walk in a natural environment (a grassland with scattered trees near the university where the study was conducted) compared to a walk in an urban area led to decreased rumination, as well as decreased activity in a region of the brain linked to rumination.

In short, there are ample reasons to spend time outdoors in natural settings. Where might you plan to spend more time to experience the satisfaction and stress relief that nature offers?

Serve Others

Self-care is anything but a selfish endeavor. The better we feel, the more we can give to others. The reverse also holds true: the more we do for others, the better we feel. Indeed, research has shown that making a point to help others leads to improvements in anxiety and depression symptoms.

Why is helping others actually self-serving? Researchers in this area have suggested several possible explanations:

1 Focusing on others can distract us from our own distress.

2 Helping others provides a sense of meaning and purpose.

3 Prosocial behaviors may cause the release of oxytocin, which is involved in trust and bonding with others.

4 There is something inherently rewarding about doing nice things for others, which may stimulate the release of dopamine.

5 Reaching out to others may lower activity in our stress response system.

There are many ways we can serve others:

- Showing support when someone we care about is struggling

- Responding with compassion when someone makes a mistake

- Taking a friend to lunch

- Making our partner's day a little easier

- Being gracious to other drivers

- Listening mindfully to another person

- Using our words to build others up

- Volunteering our time to help people in less-fortunate circumstances

- Going out of our way to help someone who can probably never repay the favor

- Donating material items we don't need to people who could use them

- Helping a neighbor with yard work

- Preparing a meal for someone in need

- Donating money to a charity whose work we find meaningful

- Visiting someone we know who's in the hospital

Helping others not only makes us happier, but also is contagious. Our helpful behaviors can multiply as others respond in kind. What opportunities can you seize this week to brighten someone's day—and your own in the process? You might even start right now.

Give Thanks

Our minds are good at focusing on what's wrong in our lives, to the exclusion of what is going well. And yet when we can notice and appreciate the good in our lives, we often find that more joy is available to us than we might have thought.

Gratitude has been linked with a wide range of positive outcomes, including better mood, lower risk for depression, less stress, greater life satisfaction, and stronger relationships. These effects can be seen even with simple, short-term gratitude practices.

For example, a team of researchers asked participants to write down either things they were thankful for or some recent hassles in their lives; the gratitude exercise led to greater positive emotion, a more positive view of one's life, and greater optimism about the future.

Gratitude also makes us more likely to help others, even at a cost to ourselves; when we realize our own coffers are full, we're more willing to share with others.

Our attentional systems are most sensitive to changes, and the things we have all the time become lost in the backdrop of our life. When we decide to practice gratitude, we're often surprised by how much we have to be thankful for. These things likely include:

- A bed of your own every night

- People in your life who care about you

- Clothes that cover your body

- A planet teeming with life

- A star to warm your planet and enable photosynthesis

- Food to nourish your body and fuel your efforts

- Electricity, running water, and climate control

- Transportation

- A relatively safe neighborhood

- Lungs that deliver oxygen to every cell in your body and get rid of carbon dioxide

- A brain that brings you all of your experiences

- A heart to pump your blood

- Your five senses

And the list goes on: things we often don't notice and appreciate until we realize we could lose them. How many times have we realized how wonderful it is simply to be healthy following a bout of illness? We can even find things to be thankful for in the midst of difficulties. For example, we might be distressed to have to take a child to the emergency room in the middle of the night, but can be grateful to have 24-hour access to medical care. A word of caution here—be careful about urging others to practice gratitude when they're going through a hard time. It can easily feel invalidating or dismissive of the struggles they're having.

There are many ways to practice gratitude, such as:

- Writing down things you are grateful for each day (doing this activity before bed can even improve sleep)

- Spending a few minutes recalling things you are thankful for

- Verbalizing your gratitude to a person in your life

- Delivering a letter to someone in which you express your gratitude to them

- Practicing gratitude meditation

Recent research suggests that *expressing* our gratitude to others is even more effective than simply reflecting on it—and may be most effective when we're feeling depressed. Take a few moments now to think about what you're grateful for in your life.

Chapter Summary and Homework

We have with us at all times a potential friend—someone who can speak to us encouragingly, praise our successes, support us when we're down, plan nice experiences for us, give us opportunities to use our strengths, and challenge us in a loving way. Unfortunately, we often play the role of our own enemy, being quick to criticize and slow to forgive ourselves, keeping ourselves from physical exercise, depriving ourselves of sleep, feeding ourselves unhealthy food, and minimizing our enjoyment in life.

Through the practices we covered in this chapter, you'll be working on a completely different approach: planning your life the way you would for someone you love. These plans will take care of your fundamental needs for nourishing food, restful sleep, and consistent movement. They also include managing the inevitable stressors you encounter and spending time in nature; finally, some of the kindest things you can do for yourself are to practice gratitude and give back to others.

These practices work well together. For example, studies of the Mediterranean lifestyle have found benefits not only of the diet but also of greater engagement in social activities and more physical activity; one study found that the Mediterranean diet alone led to about a 20 percent reduction in depression risk, whereas adding greater physical activity and more socializing led to a 50 percent reduction.

Ready to put your plans into action? You can start with these steps; focus initially on the ones that are most important to you:

1   Take stock of whether you treat yourself like someone you care about. In what ways would you like to treat yourself better?

2   Plan and start a consistent routine that prioritizes your sleep.

3   Make one positive change in your nutrition plan—for example, preparing a certain number of meals at home each week.

4 Add more movement into your day. Start slowly and build gradually.

5 Create a stress-management plan; include one small daily activity (e.g., listening to relaxing music on the way home), one bigger weekly activity (e.g., taking a yoga class), and one monthly activity (e.g., getting a professional massage).

6 Incorporate more time in nature into your week: combine time outside with social contact if possible.

7 Look for small ways to serve others every day, as well as bigger service projects to do on a regular basis (e.g., volunteering weekly at a food bank).

8 Write down three things you're grateful for every evening before you go to bed.

Conclusion: Keeping It Going

This book has presented ways to manage difficult emotions. We began with the principles of CBT and how it can be effective. We then covered the three pillars of CBT—behavioral, cognitive, and mindfulness-based techniques—and saw how these approaches can help with depression, anger, anxiety, and other emotional experiences that can overwhelm us. The previous chapter focused on being friends with ourselves, which in fact is the overarching message of CBT.

I invite you to think back to what prompted you to pick up this book. What was happening that told you it was time for a change? Review the initial goals you set during your work in chapter 2.

I hope the strategies I've offered in these chapters have helped you move toward achieving your goals. As you revisit the goals you set, what benefits have you found from the work you've done? You might talk with a loved one to see what they have noticed as you've applied the techniques from this book.

Zach thought back to how depressed he had been six months ago. He recalled how little energy and motivation he had at that time, and how irritable he'd been. He'd even started to question if he should go on living, which had startled him. From that point, he'd worked hard to reclaim his life and now stood in a very different place.

As Zach talked over these changes with his wife, Lisa, they thought together about what had made the biggest difference. "You definitely seemed happier once you started seeing friends again," Lisa said. Zach recalled how hard it'd been initially to get himself to reach out to friends and ultimately how uplifting it had been.

"I know exercise made a big difference, too," he said. He paused and then added, "I think the biggest thing was just remembering that I'm an okay person, and that people actually like me. I'd started believing really nasty things about myself."

As they continued their discussion, Zach wrote down the keys to his recovery that he wanted to remember.

Learning what helps you is one of the most important things you can discover. I strongly advise you to write down the behaviors and mind-set you need to return to in order to be at your best.

With repetition, many of these new practices will become second nature. For example, we may begin to associate certain mornings of the week with yoga or running. However, other strategies may be easier to let slide, especially those that are hard to plan specific times for—things like practicing gratitude, being present in our everyday activities, and challenging our thoughts.

Additionally, some of the challenges we face make us less likely to use the strategies that are helpful to us. For example, the hopelessness of depression might start to tell us there's "no point" in doing the very things that would make us feel better. Having a written plan makes it easier to remember the tools we need.

Zach tended to think visually, so he created an integrated plan that looked like this:

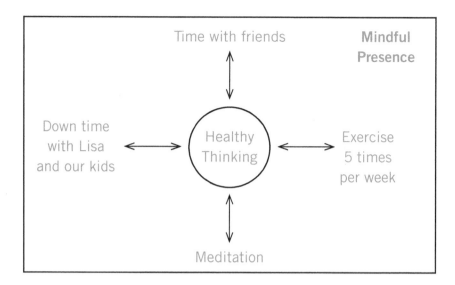

*Zach saw healthy thinking as central to feeling well and recog-
nized how his thoughts influenced his willingness to do other
things that contributed to his recovery. These activities in turn
reinforced his healthy thought patterns. He found that mindfulness had enriched each of these practices, and so framed all of
them in the context of mindful presence.*

As you summarize the strategies you found useful, think about
how they relate to each other. Notice any "virtuous circles" you've
created, in which positive changes are mutually reinforcing. For
example, exercise can make it easier to eat well, which in turn
improves your energy, making it easier to exercise.

There's no wrong format for your written plan. It just should
include the key reminders you'll need, organized in a way that will
make sense to you when you come back to it.

I also hope this book will be a resource you return to as needed.
I encourage you to take notes, underline passages, and dog-ear the
pages you'll want to review.

Even more important is the personal learning you've acquired
about what works best for you—I expect this will be your best
resource. I hope you're feeling more confident that you can

manage any difficulties you face. That knowledge alone can greatly decrease our distress.

Along with a written record of what works for you, I suggest you have an easy-to-remember phrase or slogan that captures the tools available to you. I like "Think, Act, Be," since it represents the main strategies in CBT. You might use that one or come up with your own to remind you of what's helped in the past.

What to Do If You're Still Struggling

If you haven't made the progress toward your goals that you were hoping for, you have several options.

- **Consider if you're on the right track—having made some progress—and simply have more work to do.** If that's the case, continue the things that have helped so far, and consider adding other strategies. It takes time and practice to get to a significantly better place.

- **Alternatively, it may be that this book was not the best fit for you.** Maybe your concerns were driven primarily by conflict in your marriage that requires couples therapy, or perhaps you need additional guidance from working directly with a therapist. Whatever the case may be, I encourage you to keep seeking the help you need. I've included resources in the back of this book for finding a therapist near you, as well as websites and additional books that may be helpful.

- **If at any point you find that your struggles are getting worse, not better, seek professional help right away.** You can ask for a mental health referral from your primary care doctor. I've also provided online links for finding help in the Resources section. If you think you could be a danger to yourself or someone else, go to the nearest emergency room or call 911.

Where to Go from Here?

If you're happy with the progress you've made, what's next? First, I encourage you to feel good about what you've accomplished. It takes courage and determination to persevere when life is hard, and it's no small thing to learn new skills for better living.

If you feel like you've made considerable progress toward your goals, I urge you not to limit yourself. When the worst of our difficulties is behind us, we're in a better position to ask ourselves what thriving would look like. What new goals might you set for yourself? Maybe you've been contemplating a professional move or want to make your home life better than it's ever been.

Even as you accept yourself exactly as you are, remember that growth is an ongoing process, and we can continue to raise the ceiling on our experience. Why be content with just getting by? You can use right thinking, right action, and mindful awareness not just for repairing things that are broken but for building a life you love.

STAYING WELL

It's natural when we're feeling better to stop investing as much in our well-being. I strongly recommend that you resist this tendency and keep doing the things that helped you. Now is a good time to take stock of what will be important to keep doing. I also suggest you think ahead to potential pitfalls you'll want to avoid. In the spirit of CBT, we can plan in advance for circumstances that will challenge us.

Zach knew the coming winter months not only offered fewer hours of daylight, but also made him less inclined to exercise and socialize. As the fall days grew shorter, he began to put plans in place to get him through the winter, like joining an indoor pool and scheduling time with friends.

He also talked with Lisa about his intentions for the winter
so she could support his efforts and so he would have some
accountability. Knowing he had a plan also lessened his worry
about the winter months.

What situations in your own life could lead to a setback without adequate preparation? Take some time to write down a plan for how you will handle them.

Final Thoughts

I'd like to leave you with a few key points to keep in mind.

First, remember that you're worth taking care of. Our society, for the most part, treats self-care as a self-indulgent luxury, when in fact it is not only essential for your well-being, but also benefits the people in your life.

Along those lines, I hope you surround yourself with people who care about you and bring out the best in you, and that you nurture your closest connections. Few things have as big an impact on our well-being as the quality of our relationships; strong ones will sustain you through anything that comes your way.

No matter what you're going through, make every effort to serve others. Just as self-care isn't selfish, service to others is not really self-sacrifice, and helps us the most when we're struggling.

And finally, remember to practice gratitude as often as possible, which is one of the kindest things you can do for yourself. Remind yourself of all you have, even when things are far from perfect. Gratitude doesn't deny our problems, but it does lighten their weight.

In the spirit of gratitude, I am thankful that you took the time to read this book. Keep working. Keep using your mind, your actions, and your presence to be the person you want to be. I wish you the very best as you continue your journey.

Resources

Online Resources

Visit the following online resources to enhance your learning, to find professional help, and to dive deeper into treatments and techniques.

GENERAL INFORMATION

Anxiety and Depression Association of America (ADAA)
http://www.adaa.org/understanding-anxiety
The ADAA website discusses what distinguishes normal anxiety and depression from a disorder, provides statistics about these conditions, and has information about OCD and PTSD.

Mayo Clinic Healthy Lifestyle
www.mayoclinic.org/healthy-lifestyle
The Mayo Clinic offers overviews on healthy eating, fitness, stress management, weight loss, and other topics. More in-depth articles are available under each subject heading.

National Institute of Mental Health (NIMH)
Anxiety: www.nimh.nih.gov/health/topics/anxiety-disorders/
index.shtml
Depression: www.nimh.nih.gov/health/topics/depression/
index.shtml
These websites describe common symptoms of depression and
anxiety, discuss risk factors and treatments, and discuss how to
find clinical trials you might qualify for. They also include links
to free booklets and brochures.

National Institute on Alcohol Abuse and Alcoholism (NIAAA)
www.niaaa.nih.gov
The NIAAA website provides information about the effects of
consuming alcohol, describes ongoing research trials, and includes information about clinical trials you might be eligible for. It
also includes links to free pamphlets, brochures, and fact sheets.

FINDING HELP: TREATMENT AND SUPPORT GROUPS

Anxiety and Depression Association of America (ADAA)
www.adaa.org/supportgroups
The ADAA provides information about support groups by state (as
well as some international listings), including contact information
for the support groups.

**Find a CBT Therapist—Association for Behavioral and
Cognitive Therapies (ABCT)**
www.findcbt.org
This website of the leading professional organization for CBT ther-
apists and researchers allows you to search for CBT therapists by
ZIP code, specialty, and accepted insurance.

National Alliance on Mental Illness (NAMI)

www.nami.org/Find-Support

The NAMI website offers ways to find support whether you or a loved one has a psychological disorder. Many additional resources are available on the site, including links to local NAMI chapters.

National Suicide Prevention Lifeline

www.suicidepreventionlifeline.org

1-800-273-8255

The lifeline provides free and confidential support 24 hours a day, every day of the year. Phone and online chat options are available.

Psychological Treatments—Association for Behavioral and Cognitive Therapies (ABCT)

www.abct.org/
Information/?m=mInformation&fa=_psychoTreatments

This website covers topics like evidence-based practice, treatment options, and choosing a therapist.

Research-Supported Treatments—Society of Clinical Psychology (SCP)

www.div12.org/psychological-treatments/

Division 12 of the American Psychological Association, the SCP, keeps a list of research-supported psychological treatments. The website is searchable by treatment and psychological condition.

Substance Abuse and Mental Health Services Administration (SAMHSA)

www.findtreatment.samhsa.gov/

The SAMHSA is part of the US Department of Health and Human Services and offers many resources for those who are struggling with addiction, including a treatment services locator.

MINDFULNESS

American Mindfulness Research Association (AMRA)

www.goamra.org

The AMRA presents the latest mindfulness-related research findings, as well as an interactive map for finding mindfulness training programs.

Mindfulnet

www.mindfulnet.org/index.htm

This website is a clearinghouse of information about mindfulness: what it is, how it's used, research that supports it, and more.

Books

Many of these books are on the Association for Behavioral and Cognitive Therapy's Books of Merit list, meaning they present a treatment that is based on solid research evidence. The full list can be found at **www.abct.org/SHBooks**.

ADDICTION

Anderson, Kenneth. *How to Change Your Drinking: A Harm Reduction Guide to Alcohol.*

Glasner-Edwards, Suzette. *The Addiction Recovery Skills Workbook: Changing Addictive Behaviors Using CBT, Mindfulness, and Motivational Interviewing Techniques.*

Williams, Rebecca E., and Julie S. Kraft. *The Mindfulness Workbook for Addiction: A Guide to Coping with the Grief, Stress and Anger That Trigger Addictive Behaviors.*

Wilson, Kelley, and Troy DuFrene. *The Wisdom to Know the Difference: An Acceptance and Commitment Therapy Workbook for Overcoming Substance Abuse.*

ANGER

Karmin, Aaron. *Anger Management Workbook for Men: Take Control of Your Anger and Master Your Emotions.*

McKay, Matthew, and Peter Rogers. *The Anger Control Workbook.*

Potter-Efron, Ronald. *Rage: A Step-by-Step Guide to Overcoming Explosive Anger.*

Scheff, Leonard, and Susan Edmiston. *The Cow in the Parking Lot: A Zen Approach to Overcoming Anger.*

ANXIETY

Antony, Martin M., and Richard P. Swinson. *The Shyness and Social Anxiety Workbook: Proven Techniques for Overcoming Your Fears.*

Carbonell, David. *Panic Attacks Workbook: A Guided Program for Beating the Panic Trick.*

Clark, David A., and Aaron T. Beck. *The Anxiety and Worry Workbook: The Cognitive Behavioral Solution.*

Cuncic, Arlin. *The Anxiety Workbook: A 7-Week Plan To Overcome Anxiety, Stop Worrying, and End Panic.*

Robichaud, Melisa, and Michel J. Dugas. *The Generalized Anxiety Disorder Workbook: A Comprehensive CBT Guide for Coping with Uncertainty, Worry, and Fear.*

Tolin, David. *Face Your Fears: A Proven Plan to Beat Anxiety, Panic, Phobias, and Obsessions.*

Tompkins, Michael A. *Anxiety and Avoidance: A Universal Treatment for Anxiety, Panic, and Fear.*

ASSERTIVENESS

Alberti, Robert, and Michael Emmons. *Your Perfect Right: Assertiveness and Equality in Your Life and Relationships.*

Vavrichek, Sherrie. *The Guide to Compassionate Assertiveness: How to Express Your Needs and Deal with Conflict While Keeping a Kind Heart.*

DEPRESSION

Addis, Michael E., and Christopher R. Martell. *Overcoming Depression One Step at a Time: The New Behavioral Activation Approach to Getting Your Life Back.*

Burns, David D. *The Feeling Good Handbook,* Revised edition.

Greenberger, Dennis, and Christine A. Padesky. *Mind Over Mood: Change How You Feel by Changing the Way You Think,* 2nd edition.

Joiner, Thomas Jr., and Jeremy Pettit. *The Interpersonal Solution to Depression: A Workbook for Changing How You Feel by Changing How You Relate.*

Rego, Simon and Sarah Fader. *The 10-Step Depression Relief Workbook: A Cognitive Behavioral Therapy Approach.*

DEPRESSION AND ANXIETY

Davis, Martha, Elizabeth Robbins Eshelman, and Matthew McKay. *The Relaxation and Stress Reduction Workbook,* 6th edition.

Ellis, Albert, and Robert A. Harper. *A New Guide to Rational Living.*

Gillihan, Seth J. *Retrain Your Brain: Cognitive Behavioral Therapy in 7 Weeks: A Workbook for Managing Depression and Anxiety.*

Otto, Michael, and Jasper Smits. *Exercise for Mood and Anxiety: Proven Strategies for Overcoming Depression and Enhancing Well-Being.*

MINDFULNESS

Brach, Tara. *Radical Acceptance: Embracing Your Life with the Heart of a Buddha.*

Germer, Christopher K. *The Mindful Path to Self-Compassion: Freeing Yourself from Destructive Thoughts and Emotions.*

Kabat-Zinn, Jon. *Full Catastrophe Living: Using the Wisdom of Your Body and Mind to Face Stress, Pain, and Illness,* Revised edition.

Orsillo, Susan M., and Lizabeth Roemer. *The Mindful Way Through Anxiety: Break Free from Chronic Worry and Reclaim Your Life.*

Salzberg, Sharon. *Lovingkindness: The Revolutionary Art of Happiness.*

Teasdale, John D., and Zindel V. Segal. *The Mindful Way Through Depression: Freeing Yourself from Chronic Unhappiness.*

RELATIONSHIPS

Gottman, John, and Joan DeClaire. *The Relationship Cure: A Five-Step Guide to Strengthening Your Marriage, Family, and Friendships.*

McKay, Matthew, Patrick Fanning, and Kim Paleg. *Couple Skills: Making Your Relationship Work.*

Richo, David. *How to Be an Adult in Relationships: The Five Keys to Mindful Loving.*

Ruiz, Don Miguel. *The Mastery of Love: A Practical Guide to the Art of Relationship.*

SELF-CARE

Brown, Brené. *The Gifts of Imperfection: Let Go of Who You Think You're Supposed to Be and Embrace Who You Are.*

Neff, Kristin. *Self-Compassion: The Proven Power of Being Kind to Yourself.*

SLEEP

Carney, Colleen. *Quiet Your Mind and Get to Sleep: Solutions to Insomnia for Those with Depression, Anxiety, or Chronic Pain.*

Ehrnstrom, Colleen, and Alisha L. Brosse. *End the Insomnia Struggle: A Step-by-Step Guide to Help You Get to Sleep and Stay Asleep.*

References

Akbaraly, Tasnime N., Eric J. Brunner, Jane E. Ferrie, Michael G. Marmot, Mika Kivimäki, and Archana Singh-Manoux. "Dietary Pattern and Depressive Symptoms in Middle Age." *The British Journal of Psychiatry* 195, no. 5 (October 2009): 408–413. doi: 10.1192/bjp.bp.108.058925.

Akbaraly, Tasnime N., Clarisse Kerleau, Marilyn Wyart, Nathalie Chevallier, Louise Ndiaye, Nitin Shivappa, James R. Hébert, and Mika Kivimäki. "Dietary Inflammatory Index and Recurrence of Depressive Symptoms: Results from the Whitehall II Study." *Clinical Psychological Science* 4, no. 6 (November 2016): 1125–1134. doi: 10.1177/2167702616645777.

Alcock, Ian, Mathew P. White, Benedict W. Wheeler, Lora E. Fleming, and Michael H. Depledge. "Longitudinal Effects on Mental Health of Moving to Greener and Less Green Urban Areas." *Environmental Science & Technology* 48, no. 2 (2014): 1247–1255. doi: 10.1021/es403688w.

American Psychiatric Association. *Diagnostic and Statistical Manual of Mental Disorders*, 5th ed. *(DSM-5)*. Arlington, VA: American Psychiatric Association Publishing, 2013.

Anderson, Kristen Joan. "Impulsivity, Caffeine, and Task Difficulty: A Within-Subjects Test of the Yerkes–Dodson Law." *Personality and Individual Differences* 16, no. 6 (June 1994): 813–829. doi: 10.1016/0191-8869(94)90226-7.

Arias-Carrión, Oscar, Maria Stamelou, Eric Murillo-Rodríguez, Manuel Menéndez-González, and Ernst Pöppel. "Dopaminergic Reward System:

A Short Integrative Review." *International Archives of Medicine* 3, no. 1 (2010): 24. doi: 10.1186/1755-7682-3-24.

Asmundson, Gordon J. G., Mathew G. Fetzner, Lindsey B. DeBoer, Mark B. Powers, Michael W. Otto, and Jasper A. J. Smits. "Let's Get Physical: A Contemporary Review of the Anxiolytic Effects of Exercise for Anxiety and Its Disorders." *Depression and Anxiety* 30, no. 4 (April 2013): 362–373. doi:10.1002/da.22043.

Barlow, David H., Jack M. Gorman, M. Katherine Shear, and Scott W. Woods. "Cognitive-Behavioral Therapy, Imipramine, or Their Combination for Panic Disorder: A Randomized Controlled Trial." *Journal of the American Medical Association* 283, no. 19 (2000): 2529–2536. doi: 10.1001/jama.283.19.2529.

Barth, Jürgen, Martina Schumacher, and Christoph Herrmann-Lingen. "Depression as a Risk Factor for Mortality in Patients with Coronary Heart Disease: A Meta-Analysis." *Psychosomatic Medicine* 66, no. 6 (November/December 2004): 802–813. doi: 10.1097/01.psy.0000146332.53619.b2.

Bartlett, Monica Y., and David DeSteno. "Gratitude and Prosocial Behavior: Helping When It Costs You." *Psychological Science* 17, no. 4 (April 2006): 319–325. doi: 10.1111/j.1467-9280.2006.01705.x.

Be, Daniel, Mark A. Whisman, and Lisa A. Uebelacker. "Prospective Associations Between Marital Adjustment and Life Satisfaction." *Personal Relationships* 20, no. 4 (December 2013): 728–739. doi: 10.1111/pere.12011.

Beck, Aaron T. *Cognitive Therapy and the Emotional Disorders.* New York: Penguin Books, 1979.

———. *Prisoners of Hate: The Cognitive Basis of Anger, Hostility, and Violence.* New York: HarperCollins Publishers, 1999.

Beck, Aaron T., Andrew C. Butler, Gregory K. Brown, Katherine K. Dahlsgaard, Cory F. Newman, and Judith S. Beck. "Dysfunctional Beliefs Discriminate Personality Disorders." *Behaviour Research and Therapy* 39, no. 10 (2001): 1213–1225.

Beck, Aaron T., A. John Rush, Brian F. Shaw, and Gary Emery. *Cognitive Therapy of Depression*. New York: Guilford Press, 1979.

Beck, Judith S. *Cognitive Behavior Therapy: Basics and Beyond*, 2nd ed. New York: Guilford Press, 2011.

Beck, Richard, and Ephrem Fernandez. "Cognitive-Behavioral Therapy in the Treatment of Anger: A Meta-Analysis." *Cognitive Therapy and Research* 22, no. 1 (February 1998): 63-74.

Bergmans, Rachel S., and Kristen M. Malecki. "The Association of Dietary Inflammatory Potential with Depression and Mental Well-Being Among US Adults." *Preventive Medicine* 99 (March 2017): 313-319. doi: 10.1016/j.ypmed.2017.03.016.

Bratman, Gregory N., J. Paul Hamilton, Kevin S. Hahn, Gretchen C. Daily, and James J. Gross. "Nature Experience Reduces Rumination and Subgenual Prefrontal Cortex Activation." *Proceedings of the National Academy of Sciences* 112, no. 28 (July 2015): 8567-8572. doi: /10.1073/pnas.1510459112.

Brown, Daniel K., Jo L. Barton, and Valerie F. Gladwell. "Viewing Nature Scenes Positively Affects Recovery of Autonomic Function Following Acute-Mental Stress." *Environmental Science & Technology* 47, no. 11 (June 2013): 5562-5569. doi: 10.1021/es305019p.

Brown, Emma M., Debbie M. Smith, Tracy Epton, and Christopher J. Armitage. "Do Self-Incentives Change Behavior? A Systematic Review and Meta-Analysis." *Behavior Therapy* 49, no. 1 (2018): 113-123. doi: 10.1016/j.beth.2017.09.004.

Burns, David D. *The Feeling Good Handbook*. New York: Plume/Penguin Books, 1999.

Carson, Rachel. *Silent Spring*. New York: Houghton Mifflin Harcourt, 2002.

Chiesa, Alberto, and Alessandro Serretti. "Mindfulness-Based Stress Reduction for Stress Management in Healthy People: A Review and

Meta-Analysis." *The Journal of Alternative and Complementary Medicine* 15, no. 5 (May 2009): 593–600. doi: 10.1089/acm.2008.0495.

Cooney, Gary M., Kerry Dwan, Carolyn A. Greig, Debbie A. Lawlor, Jane Rimer, Fiona R. Waugh, Marion McMurdo, and Gillian E. Mead. "Exercise for Depression." *Cochrane Database of Systematic Reviews*, no. 9 (September 2013). doi:10.1002/14651858.CD004366.pub6.

Craske, Michelle G., and David H. Barlow. *Mastery of Your Anxiety and Panic: Workbook*, 4th ed. New York: Oxford University Press, 2006.

Crocker, Jennifer, and Amy Canevello. "Creating and Undermining Social Support in Communal Relationships: The Role of Compassionate and Self-Image Goals." *Journal of Personality and Social Psychology* 95, no. 3 (September 2008): 555–575. doi: 10.1037/0022-3514.95.3.555.

Cuijpers, Pim, Tara Donker, Annemieke van Straten, J. Li, and Gerhard Andersson. "Is Guided Self-Help as Effective as Face-to-Face Psychotherapy for Depression and Anxiety Disorders? A Systematic Review and Meta-Analysis of Comparative Outcome Studies." *Psychological Medicine* 40, no. 12 (December 2010): 1943–1957. doi: 10.1017/S0033291710000772.

Davis, Daphne M., and Jeffrey A. Hayes. "What Are the Benefits of Mindfulness? A Practice Review of Psychotherapy-Related Research." *Psychotherapy* 48, no. 2 (2011): 198–208.

Derks, Daantje, and Arnold B. Bakker. "Smartphone Use, Work-Home Interference, and Burnout: A Diary Study on the Role of Recovery." *Applied Psychology* 63, no. 3 (July 2014): 411–440. doi: 10.1111/j.1464-0597.2012.00530.x.

DeRubeis, Robert J., Steven D. Hollon, Jay D. Amsterdam, Richard C. Shelton, Paula R. Young, Ronald M. Salomon, John P. O'Reardon, Margaret L. Lovett, Madeline M. Gladis, Laurel L. Brown, and Robert Gallop. "Cognitive Therapy vs Medications in the Treatment of Moderate to Severe Depression." *Archives of General Psychiatry* 62, no. 4 (2005): 409–416. doi: 10.1001/archpsyc.62.4.409.

DeRubeis, Robert J., Christian A. Webb, Tony Z. Tang, and Aaron T. Beck. "Cognitive Therapy." In *Handbook of Cognitive-Behavioral Therapies*, 3rd ed. edited by Keith S. Dobson, pp. 349–392. New York: Guilford Press, 2001.

Diamond, David M., Adam M. Campbell, Collin R. Park, Joshua Halonen, and Phillip R. Zoladz. "The Temporal Dynamics Model of Emotional Memory Processing: A Synthesis on the Neurobiological Basis of Stress-Induced Amnesia, Flashbulb and Traumatic Memories, and the Yerkes–Dodson Law." *Neural Plasticity* (2007). doi: 10.1155/2007/60803.

Division 12 of the American Psychological Association. "Research-Supported Psychological Treatments." Accessed November 15, 2017. https://www.div12.org/psychological-treatments.

Ekers, David, Lisa Webster, Annemieke Van Straten, Pim Cuijpers, David Richards, and Simon Gilbody. "Behavioural Activation for Depression: An Update of Meta-Analysis of Effectiveness and Sub Group Analysis." *PloS One* 9, no. 6 (June 2014): e100100. doi: 10.1371/journal.pone.0100100.

Ellenbogen, Jeffrey M., Jessica D. Payne, and Robert Stickgold. "The Role of Sleep in Declarative Memory Consolidation: Passive, Permissive, Active or None?" *Current Opinion in Neurobiology* 16, no. 6 (December 2006): 716–722. doi: 10.1016/j.conb.2006.10.006.

Ellis, Albert. *Reason and Emotion in Psychotherapy.* Secaucus, NJ: Citadel Press, 1962.

Emmons, Robert A., and Michael E. McCullough. "Counting Blessings Versus Burdens: An Experimental Investigation of Gratitude and Subjective Well-Being in Daily Life." *Journal of Personality and Social Psychology* 84, no. 2 (February 2003): 377–389.

Erickson, Thane M., M. Teresa Granillo, Jennifer Crocker, James L. Abelson, Hannah E. Reas, and Christina M. Quach. "Compassionate and Self-Image Goals as Interpersonal Maintenance Factors in Clinical Depression and Anxiety." *Journal of Clinical Psychology* (September 2017) doi: 10.1002/jclp.22524.

Felmingham, Kim, Andrew Kemp, Leanne Williams, Pritha Das, Gerard Hughes, Anthony Peduto, and Richard Bryant. "Changes in Anterior Cingulate and Amygdala After Cognitive Behavior Therapy of Posttraumatic Stress Disorder." *Psychological Science* 18, no. 2 (February 2007): 127–129.

Fox, Jesse, and Jennifer J. Moreland. "The Dark Side of Social Networking Sites: An Exploration of the Relational and Psychological Stressors Associated with Facebook Use and Affordances." *Computers in Human Behavior* 45 (April 2015): 168–176. doi: 10.1016/j.chb.2014.11.083.

Francis, Kylie, and Michel J. Dugas. "Assessing Positive Beliefs About Worry: Validation of a Structured Interview." *Personality and Individual Differences* 37, no. 2 (July 2004): 405–415. doi: 10.1016/j.paid.2003.09.012.

Gillihan, Seth J., John A. Detre, Martha J. Farah, and Hengyi Rao. "Neural Substrates Associated with Weather-Induced Mood Variability: An Exploratory Study Using ASL Perfusion fMRI." *Journal of Cognitive Science* 12, no. 2 (2011): 195–210.

Gillihan, Seth J., Hengyi Rao, Jiongjiong Wang, John A. Detre, Jessica Breland, Geena Mary V. Sankoorikal, Edward S. Brodkin, and Martha J. Farah. "Serotonin Transporter Genotype Modulates Amygdala Activity During Mood Regulation." *Social Cognitive and Affective Neuroscience* 5, no. 1 (March 2010): 1–10. doi: 10.1093/scan/nsp035.

Gillihan, Seth J., Chenjie Xia, Alisa A. Padon, Andrea S. Heberlein, Martha J. Farah, and Lesley K. Fellows. "Contrasting Roles for Lateral and Ventromedial Prefrontal Cortex in Transient and Dispositional Affective Experience." *Social Cognitive and Affective Neuroscience* 6, no. 1 (January 2011): 128–137. doi: 10.1093/scan/nsq026.

Grant, Adam. *Originals: How Non-Conformists Move the World.* New York: Penguin, 2017.

Grant, Joshua A., Emma G. Duerden, Jérôme Courtemanche, Mariya Cherkasova, Gary H. Duncan, and Pierre Rainville. "Cortical Thickness,

Mental Absorption and Meditative Practice: Possible Implications for Disorders of Attention." *Biological Psychology* 92, no. 2 (2013): 275–281.

Hartig, Terry, Richard Mitchell, Sjerp De Vries, and Howard Frumkin. "Nature and Health." *Annual Review of Public Health* 35 (2014): 207–228. doi: 10.1146/annurev-publhealth-032013-182443.

Hellström, Kerstin, and Lars-Göran Öst. "One-Session Therapist Directed Exposure vs Two Forms of Manual Directed Self-Exposure in the Treatment of Spider Phobia." *Behaviour Research and Therapy* 33, no. 8 (November 1995): 959–965. doi: 1016/0005-7967(95)00028-V.

Hirshkowitz, Max, Kaitlyn Whiton, Steven M. Albert, Cathy Alessi, Oliviero Bruni, Lydia DonCarlos, Nancy Hazen, et al. "National Sleep Foundation's Sleep Time Duration Recommendations: Methodology and Results Summary." *Sleep Health* 1, no. 1 (2015): 40–43. doi: 10.1016/j.sleh.2014.12.010.

Hofmann, Stefan G., Anu Asnaani, Imke J. J. Vonk, Alice T. Sawyer, and Angela Fang. "The Efficacy of Cognitive Behavioral Therapy: A Review of Meta-Analyses." *Cognitive Therapy and Research* 36, no. 5 (October 2012): 427–440. doi: 10.1007/s10608-012-9476-1.

Hofmann, Stefan G., Alice T. Sawyer, Ashley A. Witt, and Diana Oh. "The Effect of Mindfulness-Based Therapy on Anxiety and Depression: A Meta-Analytic Review." *Journal of Consulting and Clinical Psychology* 78, no. 2 (April 2010): 169–183. doi: 10.1037/a0018555.

Hollon, Steven D., Robert J. DeRubeis, Richard C. Shelton, Jay D. Amsterdam, Ronald M. Salomon, John P. O'Reardon, Margaret L. Lovett, et al. "Prevention of Relapse Following Cognitive Therapy vs Medications in Moderate to Severe Depression." *Archives of General Psychiatry* 62, no. 4 (April 2005): 417–422. doi: 10.1001/archpsyc.62.4.417.

Irwin, Michael R., Minge Wang, Capella O. Campomayor, Alicia Collado-Hidalgo, and Steve Cole. "Sleep Deprivation and Activation of Morning Levels of Cellular and Genomic Markers of Inflammation."

Archives of Internal Medicine 166, no. 16 (2006): 1756–1762. doi: 10.1001/archinte.166.16.1756.

Jacka, Felice N., Julie A. Pasco, Arnstein Mykletun, Lana J. Williams, Allison M. Hodge, Sharleen Linette O'Reilly, Geoffrey C. Nicholson, Mark A. Kotowicz, and Michael Berk. "Association of Western and Traditional Diets with Depression and Anxiety in Women." *American Journal of Psychiatry* 167, no. 3 (March 2010): 305–311. doi: 10.1176/appi.ajp.2009.09060881.

James, William. *On Vital Reserves: The Energies of Men. The Gospel of Relaxation*. New York: Henry Holt and Company, 1911.

Jeanne, Miranda, James J. Gross, Jacqueline B. Persons, and Judy Hahn. "Mood Matters: Negative Mood Induction Activates Dysfunctional Attitudes in Women Vulnerable to Depression." *Cognitive Therapy and Research* 22, no. 4 (August 1998): 363–376. doi: 10.1023/A:1018709212986.

Kabat-Zinn, Jon, Leslie Lipworth, and Robert Burney. "The Clinical Use of Mindfulness Meditation for the Self-Regulation of Chronic Pain." *Journal of Behavioral Medicine* 8, no. 2 (1985): 163–190.

Kaplan, Bonnie J., Julia J. Rucklidge, Amy Romijn, and Kevin McLeod. "The Emerging Field of Nutritional Mental Health: Inflammation, the Microbiome, Oxidative Stress, and Mitochondrial Function." *Clinical Psychological Science* 3, no. 6 (2015): 964–980.

Kessler, Ronald C., Patricia Berglund, Olga Demler, Robert Jin, Doreen Koretz, Kathleen R. Merikangas, A. John Rush, Ellen E. Walters, and Philip S. Wang. "The Epidemiology of Major Depressive Disorder: Results from the National Comorbidity Survey Replication (NCS-R)." *Journal of the American Medical Association* 289, no. 23 (June 2003): 3095–3105. doi: 10.1001/jama.289.23.3095.

Kessler, Ronald C., Patricia Berglund, Olga Demler, Robert Jin, Kathleen R. Merikangas, and Ellen E. Walters. "Lifetime Prevalence and Age-of-Onset Distributions of *DSM-IV* Disorders in the National

Comorbidity Survey Replication." *Archives of General Psychiatry* 62, no. 6 (June 2005): 593–602. doi: 10.1001/archpsyc.62.6.593.

Kessler, Ronald C., Wai Tat Chiu, Robert Jin, Ayelet Meron Ruscio, Katherine Shear, and Ellen E. Walters. "The Epidemiology of Panic Attacks, Panic Disorder, and Agoraphobia in the National Comorbidity Survey Replication." *Archives of General Psychiatry* 63, no. 4 (April 2006): 415–424. doi:10.1001/archpsyc.63.4.415.

Kessler, Ronald C., Maria Petukhova, Nancy A. Sampson, Alan M. Zaslavsky, and Hans Ullrich Wittchen. "Twelve-Month and Lifetime Prevalence and Lifetime Morbid Risk of Anxiety and Mood Disorders in the United States." *International Journal of Methods in Psychiatric Research* 21, no. 3 (September 2012): 169–184. doi:10.1002/mpr.1359.

Kessler, Ronald C., Ayelet Meron Ruscio, Katherine Shear, and Hans-Ulrich Wittchen. "Epidemiology of Anxiety Disorders." In *Behavioral Neurobiology of Anxiety and Its Treatment*, edited by Murray B. Stein and Thomas Steckler, pp. 21–35. Heidelberg, Germany: Springer, 2009.

Krogh, Jesper, Merete Nordentoft, Jonathan A. C. Sterne, and Debbie A. Lawlor. "The Effect of Exercise in Clinically Depressed Adults: Systematic Review and Meta-Analysis of Randomized Controlled Trials." *The Journal of Clinical Psychiatry* 72, no. 4 (April 2011): 529–538. doi: 10.4088/JCP.08r04913blu.

Kross, Ethan, Philippe Verduyn, Emre Demiralp, Jiyoung Park, David Seungjae Lee, Natalie Lin, Holly Shablack, John Jonides, and Oscar Ybarra. "Facebook Use Predicts Declines in Subjective Well-Being in Young Adults." *PloS One* 8, no. 8 (August 2013): e69841. doi: 10.1371/journal.pone.0069841.

Lai, Jun S., Sarah Hiles, Alessandra Bisquera, Alexis J. Hure, Mark McEvoy, and John Attia. "A Systematic Review and Meta-Analysis of Dietary Patterns and Depression in Community-Dwelling Adults." *The American Journal of Clinical Nutrition* 99, no. 1 (January 2014): 181–197. doi: 10.3945/ajcn.113.06988.

LeDoux, Joseph E. "Emotion: Clues from the Brain." *Annual Review of Psychology* 46, no. 1 (1995): 209–235.

Lejuez, C. W., Derek R. Hopko, Ron Acierno, Stacey B. Daughters, and Sherry L. Pagoto. "Ten-Year Revision of the Brief Behavioral Activation Treatment for Depression: Revised Treatment Manual." *Behavior Modification* 35, no. 2 (February 2011): 111–161.

Locke, Edwin A., and Gary P. Latham. "Building a Practically Useful Theory of Goal Setting and Task Motivation: A 35-Year Odyssey." *American Psychologist* 57, no. 9 (2002): 705–717. doi: 10.1037/0003-066X.57.9.705.

Ma, S. Helen, and John D. Teasdale. "Mindfulness-Based Cognitive Therapy for Depression: Replication and Exploration of Differential Relapse Prevention Effects." *Journal of Consulting and Clinical Psychology* 72, no. 1 (February 2004): 31–40. doi: 10.1037/0022-006X.72.1.31.

Minkel, Jared D., Siobhan Banks, Oo Htaik, Marisa C. Moreta, Christopher W. Jones, Eleanor L. McGlinchey, Norah S. Simpson, and David F. Dinges. "Sleep Deprivation and Stressors: Evidence for Elevated Negative Affect in Response to Mild Stressors When Sleep Deprived." *Emotion* 12, no. 5 (October 2012): 1015–1020. doi: 10.1037/a0026871.

Mitchell, Matthew D., Philip Gehrman, Michael Perlis, and Craig A. Umscheid. "Comparative Effectiveness of Cognitive Behavioral Therapy for Insomnia: A Systematic Review." *BMC Family Practice* 13 (May 2012): 1–11. doi: 10.1186/1471-2296-13-40.

Nelson, Julia, and Allison G. Harvey. "An Exploration of Pre Sleep Cognitive Activity in Insomnia: Imagery and Verbal Thought." *British Journal of Clinical Psychology* 42, no. 3 (September 2003): 271–288.

Nemeroff, Charles B., J. Douglas Bremner, Edna B. Foa, Helen S. Mayberg, Carol S. North, and Murray B. Stein. "Posttraumatic Stress Disorder: A State-of-the-Science Review." *Journal of Psychiatric Research* 40, no. 1 (2006): 1–21. doi: 10.1016/j.jpsychires.2005.07.005.

National Institute of Mental Health. "Mental Health Medications." Accessed November 21, 2017. https://www.nimh.nih.gov/health/topics /mental-health-medications/index.shtml.

National Institute of Mental Health. "Mental Health Statistics." Accessed November 10, 2017. https://www.nimh.nih.gov/health/topics/index.shtml.

O'Connell, Brenda H., Deirdre O'Shea, and Stephen Gallagher. "Feeling Thanks and Saying Thanks: A Randomized Controlled Trial Examining If and How Socially Oriented Gratitude Journals Work." *Journal of Clinical Psychology* 73, no. 10 (October 2017): 1280–1300. doi: 10.1002/jclp.22469.

Opie, R. S., C. Itsiopoulos, N. Parletta, A. Sánchez-Villegas, T. N. Akbaraly, Anu Ruusunen, and F. N. Jacka. "Dietary Recommendations for the Prevention of Depression." *Nutritional Neuroscience* 20, no. 3 (April 2017): 161–171. doi: 10.1179/1476830515Y.0000000043.

Öst, Lars-Göran. "One-Session Treatment of Specific Phobias." *Behaviour Research and Therapy* 27, no. 1 (February 1989): 1–7. doi: 10.1016/0005 -7967(89)90113-7.

Owen, John M. "Transdiagnostic Cognitive Processes in High Trait Anger." *Clinical Psychology Review* 31, no. 2 (2011): 193–202. doi: 10.1016 /j.cpr.2010.10.003.

Parletta, Natalie, Dorota Zarnowiecki, Jihyun Cho, Amy Wilson, Svetlana Bogomolova, Anthony Villani, Catherine Itsiopoulos, et al. "A Mediterranean-Style Dietary Intervention Supplemented with Fish Oil Improves Diet Quality and Mental Health in People with Depression: A Randomized Controlled Trial (HELFIMED)." *Nutritional Neuroscience* (2017): 1–14.

Piet, Jacob, and Esben Hougaard. "The Effect of Mindfulness-Based Cognitive Therapy for Prevention of Relapse in Recurrent Major Depressive Disorder: A Systematic Review and Meta-Analysis." *Clinical Psychology Review* 31, no. 6 (August 2011): 1032–1040. doi: 10.1016/j.cpr.2011.05.002.

Psychology Today. "Agoraphobia." Accessed February 10, 2017. https://www.psychologytoday.com/conditions/agoraphobia.

Rahe, Corinna, and Klaus Berger. "Nutrition and Depression: Current Evidence on the Association of Dietary Patterns with Depression and Its Subtypes." In *Cardiovascular Diseases and Depression*, pp. 279-304. Springer International Publishing, 2016.

Rao, Hengyi, Seth J. Gillihan, Jiongjiong Wang, Marc Korczykowski, Geena Mary V. Sankoorikal, Kristin A. Kaercher, Edward S. Brodkin, John A. Detre, and Martha J. Farah. "Genetic Variation in Serotonin Transporter Alters Resting Brain Function in Healthy Individuals." *Biological Psychiatry* 62, no. 6 (2007): 600-606. doi: 10.1016/j.biopsych.2006.11.028.

Raposa, Elizabeth B., Holly B. Laws, and Emily B. Ansell. "Prosocial Behavior Mitigates the Negative Effects of Stress in Everyday Life." *Clinical Psychological Science* 4, no. 4 (2016): 691-698.

Rotenstein, Aliza, Harry Z. Davis, and Lawrence Tatum. "Early Birds Versus Just-in-Timers: The Effect of Procrastination on Academic Performance of Accounting Students." *Journal of Accounting Education* 27, no. 4 (2009): 223-232. doi: 10.1016/j.jaccedu.2010.08.001.

Rucklidge, Julia J., and Bonnie J. Kaplan. "Nutrition and Mental Health." *Clinical Psychological Science* 4, no. 6 (2016): 1082-1084.

Saini, Michael. "A Meta-Analysis of the Psychological Treatment of Anger: Developing Guidelines for Evidence-Based Practice." *Journal of the American Academy of Psychiatry and the Law Online* 37, no. 4 (2009): 473-488.

Salzman, C. Daniel, and Stefano Fusi. "Emotion, Cognition, and Mental State Representation in Amygdala and Prefrontal Cortex." *Annual Review of Neuroscience* 33 (2010): 173-202. doi: 10.1146/annurev.neuro.051508.135256.

Sánchez-Villegas, Almudena, Miguel Ruíz-Canela, Alfredo Gea, Francisca Lahortiga, and Miguel A. Martínez-González. "The Association Between the Mediterranean Lifestyle and Depression." *Clinical Psychological Science* 4, no. 6 (2016): 1085-1093.

Sapolsky, Robert M. *Why Zebras Don't Get Ulcers: The Acclaimed Guide to Stress, Stress-Related Diseases, and Coping.* New York: Holt Paperbacks, 2004.

Segal, Zindel V., Michael Gemar, and Susan Williams. "Differential Cognitive Response to a Mood Challenge Following Successful Cognitive Therapy or Pharmacotherapy for Unipolar Depression." *Journal of Abnormal Psychology* 108, no. 1 (1999): 3–10. doi: 10.1037/0021-843X .108.1.3.

Seligman, Martin E. P., Tayyab Rashid, and Acacia C. Parks. "Positive Psychotherapy." *American Psychologist* 61, no. 8 (2006): 774–788. doi: 10.1037/0003-066X.61.8.774.

Selye, Hans. "A Syndrome Produced by Diverse Nocuous Agents." *Nature* 138, no. 32 (July 1936). doi: 10.1038/138032a0.

Stathopoulou, Georgia, Mark B. Powers, Angela C. Berry, Jasper A. J. Smits, and Michael W. Otto. "Exercise Interventions for Mental Health: A Quantitative and Qualitative Review." *Clinical Psychology: Science and Practice* 13, no. 2 (May 2006): 179–193. doi: 10.1111/j.1468-2850.2006 .00021.x.

Sugiyama, Takemi, Eva Leslie, Billie Giles-Corti, and Neville Owen. "Associations of Neighbourhood Greenness with Physical and Mental Health: Do Walking, Social Coherence and Local Social Interaction Explain the Relationships?" *Journal of Epidemiology and Community Health* 62, no. 5 (2008): e9.

Tang, Tony Z., and Robert J. DeRubeis. "Sudden Gains and Critical Sessions in Cognitive-Behavioral Therapy for Depression." *Journal of Consulting and Clinical Psychology* 67, no. 6 (1999): 894–904.

Tang, Tony Z., Robert J. DeRubeis, Steven D. Hollon, Jay Amsterdam, and Richard Shelton. "Sudden Gains in Cognitive Therapy of Depression and Depression Relapse/Recurrence." *Journal of Consulting and Clinical Psychology* 75, no. 3 (2007): 404–408. doi: 10.1037/0022-006X.75.3.404.

Teasdale, John D., Zindel Segal, and J. Mark G. Williams. "How Does Cognitive Therapy Prevent Depressive Relapse and Why Should Attentional Control (Mindfulness) Training Help?" *Behaviour Research and Therapy* 33, no. 1 (January 1995): 25-39.

Teasdale, John D., Zindel V. Segal, J. Mark G. Williams, Valerie A. Ridgeway, Judith M. Soulsby, and Mark A. Lau. "Prevention of Relapse/Recurrence in Major Depression by Mindfulness-Based Cognitive Therapy." *Journal of Consulting and Clinical Psychology* 68, no. 4 (2000): 615-623. doi: 10.1037//0022-006X.68.4.615.

Thimm, Jens C. "Personality and Early Maladaptive Schemas: A Five-Factor Model Perspective." *Journal of Behavior Therapy and Experimental Psychiatry* 41, no. 4 (2010): 373-380. doi: 10.1016/j.jbtep.2010.03.009.

Tice, Dianne M., and Roy F. Baumeister. "Longitudinal Study of Procrastination, Performance, Stress, and Health: The Costs and Benefits of Dawdling." *Psychological Science* 8, no. 6 (1997): 454-458.

Tolin, David F. "Is Cognitive-Behavioral Therapy More Effective Than Other Therapies? A Meta-Analytic Review." *Clinical Psychology Review* 30, no. 6 (August 2010): 710-720. doi: 10.1016/j.cpr.2010.05.003.

Trungpa, Chögyam. *Shambhala: The Sacred Path of the Warrior.* Boston: Shambhala, 2007.

Vogel, Erin A., Jason P. Rose, Lindsay R. Roberts, and Katheryn Eckles. "Social Comparison, Social Media, and Self-Esteem." *Psychology of Popular Media Culture* 3, no. 4 (2014): 206-222. doi: 10.1037/ppm0000047.

Walsh, Roger. "Lifestyle and Mental Health." *American Psychologist* 66, no. 7 (2011): 579-592. doi: 10.1037/a0021769.

Watters, Paul Andrew, Frances Martin, and Zoltan Schreter. "Caffeine and Cognitive Performance: The Nonlinear Yerkes-Dodson Law." *Human Psychopharmacology: Clinical and Experimental* 12, no. 3 (1997): 249-257. doi: 10.1002/(SICI)1099-1077(199705/06)12:3<249::AID-HUP865>3.0.CO;2-J.

Winbush, Nicole Y., Cynthia R. Gross, and Mary Jo Kreitzer. "The Effects of Mindfulness-Based Stress Reduction on Sleep Disturbance: A Systematic Review." *Explore: The Journal of Science and Healing* 3, no. 6 (2007): 585-591. doi: 10.1016/j.explore.2007.08.003.

Wise, Roy A. "Dopamine, Learning and Motivation." *Nature Reviews Neuroscience* 5, no. 6 (2004): 483-494. doi: 10.1038/nrn1406.

Wood, Alex M., Jeffrey J. Froh, and Adam W. A. Geraghty. "Gratitude and Well-Being: A Review and Theoretical Integration." *Clinical Psychology Review* 30, no. 7 (2010): 890-905. doi: 10.1016/j.cpr.2010.03.005.

Wright, Steven, Andrew Day, and Kevin Howells. "Mindfulness and the Treatment of Anger Problems." *Aggression and Violent Behavior* 14, no. 5 (2009): 396-401. doi: 10.1016/j.avb.2009.06.008.

Index

A

Acceptance, 89-90, 100, 137, 154
Acceptance and Commitment Therapy (ACT), 91-92
Acceptance-Based Behavioral Therapy, 92
Accountability, 47
Acting (behavioral)
    anger strategies, 152-153
    procrastination strategies, 111-114
    Think Act Be framework, 8, 108
    worry, fear, and anxiety
        strategies, 133-135
Activities. See also Values
    effective approaches, 45-48
    identifying, 39-42
    tracking, 48-49, 50-51
Acute stress, 14
Agoraphobia, 126
Alcock, Ian, 174
Alcohol consumption, 25-26
Amygdala, 29, 130
Anger
    about, 14-15
    behavioral strategies for, 152-153
    benefits of, 145-146
    cognitive strategies for, 148-152
    excessive, 147
    managing, 149
    meditation for, 156
    mindfulness strategies for, 153-155
    and thoughts, 63
    understanding, 143-145

Anxiety
    about, 11-12, 121-123
    behavioral strategies for, 133-135
    and the brain, 130-131
    cognitive strategies for, 129, 131-133
    mindfulness strategies for, 135-137
    and thoughts, 63
Assumptions, 151
Avoidance, 33-34, 109, 126, 127. See also Behavioral activation
Awareness, 96-97, 98-99, 168-169

B

Beck, Aaron T., 3, 4, 56-57, 153
Beck, Judith S., 71, 83
"Beginner's mind," 97
Behavioral activation
    applying to goals, 43-44
    effective approaches, 45-48
    motivation, 34-35
    strategies for meeting goals, 35-42
    and values, 39
Behavioral therapy, 3, 4
Being (mindfulness)
    anger strategies, 153-155
    procrastination
        strategies, 114-115, 117-118
    Think Act Be framework, 8, 108
    worry, fear, and anxiety
        strategies, 135-137
Benzodiazepines, 9
Biased thinking, 54, 147
Black-and-white thinking, 56

Breathing, 135-136, 155
Burns, David D., 56-57

C

Catastrophizing, 56
CBT. *See* Cognitive behavioral
    therapy (CBT)
Chronic stress, 14
Cirillo, Francesco, 113
Cognitive behavioral therapy (CBT)
    development of, 2-5
    how it works, 8, 10
    principles of, 5-8
Cognitive behavioral therapy for
    insomnia (CBT-I), 163
Cognitive distortions, 56-57
Cognitive therapy, 3-4
Compassion, 21, 45
Compulsions, 127-128
"Coping card," 83
Core beliefs
    building new, 78-84
    defined, 71
    identifying, 73-76
    origins of, 76-78
    reasons for, 72-73
"Cycling the puck," 81

D

Depersonalization, 125
Depression, 10, 11, 29, 33, 63, 91.
    See also Behavioral
    activation
Derealization, 125
DeRubeis, Rob, 81
Diet, and mental health, 26, 164-166
Discomfort, 115
Discounting the positive, 56
Dodson, John, 123
Domestic tasks, 27
"Downward arrow technique," 61-62
Drug use, 25-26

E

Education, 24
Ellis, Albert, 3
Emotional reasoning, 56
Emotions, 92. *See also* Core beliefs;
    Thoughts; *specific emotions*
Entitlement, 57
Exercise, 25, 102, 166-167
Exposure and response
    prevention, 128
Exposure therapy, 133-134, 137-140

F

Faith, 23-24
False sense of helplessness, 57
False sense of responsibility, 57
Farah, Martha, 30
Fear. *See also* Exposure therapy
    about, 120, 121, 128-129
    behavioral strategies for, 133-135
    cognitive strategies for, 129, 131-133
    mindfulness strategies for, 135-137
Fortune telling, 57
Freud, Sigmund, 3

G

Generalized anxiety disorder
    (GAD), 13, 92, 126
Goals
    behavioral activation
        applications, 43-44
    behavioral activation
        strategies, 35-42
    benefits of, 19
    identifying strengths, 20, 22-28
    importance of, 6
    lack of progress towards, 185
    and mindfulness, 100
    principles for setting, 19-20, 21
    realistic, 21
Grant, Adam, 107
Gratitude, 176-178, 187

H

Habits, 158–160
Hayes, Steven, 91
Hippocampus, 30, 130
Hopelessness, 63
Household labor, 27
Hyperarousal, 127
Hypothalamus, 29, 130

I

Inflammation, 165
Injustice, 63
Insomnia, 162–163
Internet, 116
Irritability, 146

J

Joy, 40

K

Kabat-Zinn, Jon, 5, 101

L

Lazarus, Arnold, 3
Leisure time, 27–28
Limbic system, 28–30, 130–131

M

Major depressive disorder, 29
Meaning, 23–24
Medications, 9
Meditation
    for anger management, 156
    how to start, 94–96
    and mindfulness, 100–101
    and procrastination, 115
    sitting, 93
    types of, 93

Mediterranean diet, 164–165, 179
Mind-body connection, 24–25
Mindful awareness, 96–97, 98–99
Mindfulness
    about, 5, 87
    benefits of, 91–92
    myths, 97, 99–101
    practicing, 93–94
    strategies for procrastination,
        114–115, 117–118
    strategies for worry, fear, and
        anxiety, 135–137
Mindfulness-based cognitive therapy
    (MBCT), 91
Mindfulness-based stress reduction
    (MBSR), 5, 101
Mindful walking, 102
Mind reading, 57
Mood disorders, 15. See also specific
Motivation, 123, 146

N

National Suicide Prevention
    Lifeline, 10
Nature, 174–175
Negative automatic thoughts, 7, 53.
    See also Core beliefs; Thoughts
Negative reinforcement, 107, 128
Nervous system
    parasympathetic, 155, 168, 174
    sympathetic, 14, 130, 168
Neuroticism, 76
Nutrition, 26, 164–166

O

Observation, 155
Obsessions, 127–128
Obsessive-compulsive disorder
    (OCD), 124, 127–128
Orsillo, Susan, 92
Outsourcing happiness, 57
Overgeneralization, 56

P

Panic, 12–13
Panic attacks, 125–126
Panic disorder, 125–126
Parasympathetic nervous
    system, 55, 168, 174
Perfectionism, 113
Personalization, 57
Phobias, 124
Physical health, 24–27
Pituitary gland, 130
Pomodoro technique, 113
Positive reinforcement, 107, 114
Posttraumatic stress disorder
    (PTSD), 29, 124, 126–127
Prediction testing, 133
Prefrontal cortex, 29, 30
Presence, 88–89, 115, 136
Procrastination
    behavioral strategies for, 111–114
    being on time, 110–111
    benefits of, 107
    characteristics of, 105
    cognitive strategies for, 108–109, 111
    internet-based, 116
    mindfulness strategies
        for, 114–115, 117–118
    reasons for, 106–107
Progressive muscle relaxation, 170–172
Projection, 73
Psychoanalysis, 3

R

Real-world engagement, 172–173
Recreation, 27–28
Relapse, 6–7
Relationships, 22–23
Relaxation, 27–28, 155, 170–172
Religion, 97, 99
Roemer, Lizabeth, 92
Routines, 7
Rumination, 147, 150, 154

S

Safety behaviors, 134–135
Schemas, 72
Scripts, 72
Segal, Zindel, 5, 91
Selective attention, 147
Selective serotonin reuptake inhibitors
    (SSRIs), 9
Selye, Hans, 168
Serving others, 175–176
Shoulding, 56, 150
Sitting meditation, 93
Sleep, 27, 152, 160–164
Smoking, 25–26
Social anxiety, 12
Social anxiety disorder, 124–125
Stress, 13–14, 168–169
"Sudden gains," 81
Suicidal thoughts, 10
Sympathetic nervous system, 14,
    130, 168

T

Teasdale, John, 91
Technology, 116, 172–173
Think Act Be framework, 8, 108, 119,
    185. See also Acting (behavioral);
    Being (mindfulness); Thinking
    (cognitive)
Thinking (cognitive)
    anger strategies, 148–152
    procrastination strategies, 108–119
    Think Act Be framework, 8, 108
    worry, fear, and anxiety
        strategies, 129, 131–133
Thinking errors, 56–57
Thoughts. See also Core beliefs
    breaking negative thought
        patterns, 64–69
    common themes in, 63
    "downward arrow technique," 61–62
    identifying problematic, 55, 58
    negative automatic, 7, 53
    power of, 53–54

recording, 58–62
thinking errors, 56–57
Threat, 63
Tobacco use, 25–26
To-do lists, 117–118
Triggers, 148
Tuckman, Ari, 116, 117

U

Uncertainty, 137

V

Values, 35–39. *See also* Activities
"Virtuous avoidance," 109
"Virtuous circles," 11, 184

W

Williams, Mark, 91
Wolpe, Joseph, 3
Work, 24
Worry
    about, 13, 121
    behavioral strategies for, 133–135
    cognitive strategies for, 129, 131–133
    mindfulness strategies for, 135–137

Y

Yerkes, Robert, 123
Yoga, 93

Acknowledgments

Many people contributed in one way or another to the writing of this book. Appreciation goes first to my parents, Charles and Carolyn Gillihan, for all their work in raising five sons. It wasn't until I'd been out of the house for a couple decades that I understood what it takes to be a loving and involved parent while dealing with the best and hardest parts of life. I also thank my brothers, Yonder, Malachi, Tim, and Charlie—life would not be the same without the bond we share.

I started my clinical training at The George Washington University and was lucky to have Dr. Raymond Pasi teach my first course. I've continued to benefit from his wisdom and humor over the past 17 years. Professor Rich Lanthier introduced me to the field of human development and was instrumental in guiding my own development in graduate school.

I was drawn to the University of Pennsylvania for my doctorate because of its strong reputation for CBT training and had an even better experience than I'd hoped for thanks to the talented faculty. Dr. Dianne Chambless, a leader in evidence-based psychological treatments, enriched my experience through her role as Director of Clinical Training. Dr. Melissa Hunt taught me skills in evidence-based assessment that I continue to rely on. Dr. Alan Goldstein, my first therapy supervisor, proved that CBT can be as warm as it is effective. I enjoyed Dr. Rob DeRubeis's cognitive therapy supervision so much that I completed his practicum three times, and I strive to reflect his approach in my own role as supervisor. My brilliant thesis advisor Dr. Martha Farah made my graduate experience a rich one; I continue to benefit from her kindness and guidance.

Thanks also to Dr. Zindel Segal, pioneer of mindfulness-based cognitive therapy, for a stimulating introduction to mindfulness in a clinical context toward the end of my graduate training.

Dr. Elyssa Kushner helped me build on that introduction when I was in my first faculty position; her instruction in mindfulness-based treatment for anxiety provided an invaluable "third wave" in my own development as a therapist. I learned from Dr. Edna Foa not only the nuances of powerful exposure treatments, but also how to make each word count as a writer; her passion for dissemination is reflected in my work after leaving full-time academia.

Since that time, I've been most fortunate to connect with a strong and talented group of clinicians in the community, including my frequent collaborators Drs. Rick Summers, David Steinman, Donald Tavakoli, Pace Duckett, Matt Kayser, Dhwani Shah, Catherine Riley, Teresa Saris, and Madeleine Weiser (who also provides stellar pediatric care to our kids), along with others too numerous to list here.

I'm grateful for the support and collegiality of my friends and fellow psychologists Drs. Lucy Faulconbridge, Jesse Suh, David Yusko, Steven Tsao, Mitch Greene, Marc Tannenbaum, Eliot Garson, Katherine Dahlsgaard, and others. I have also benefited enormously from my friendships with sleep specialist Dr. Jeff Ellenbogen, psychiatrists Dr. Matt Hurford and Dr. Ted Brodkin, and fitness and weight-loss specialist Dr. Aria Campbell-Danesh. Thanks to wellness expert Dr. James Kelley for stimulating discussions about the place of CBT in overall well-being, not to mention countless commiseration sessions on our early morning runs—I miss those times.

I continue to benefit from the expertise and counsel of Corey Field. Thank you to my fantastic editor at Callisto Media, Nana K. Twumasi, for the opportunity to work together again.

Over the past two decades, I've had the privilege of treating hundreds of men and women who were bold enough to reach out for help. Thank you for allowing me to share part of your journey—many of the lessons I've learned along the way are captured in this book.

Finally, my deepest gratitude as always goes to my wife, Marcia, and our three children. You are a continual source of love and inspiration in everything I do. Words can't describe how fortunate I feel to share life's adventure with you.

About the Author

Licensed psychologist **Seth J. Gillihan, PhD**, is a Clinical Assistant Professor of Psychology in the Psychiatry Department at the University of Pennsylvania. Dr. Gillihan has written more than 40 journal articles and book chapters on the effectiveness of cognitive behavioral therapy (CBT) for anxiety and depression, how CBT works, and the use of brain imaging to study psychiatric conditions. He is the author of *Retrain Your Brain: Cognitive Behavioral Therapy in 7 Weeks*, a self-directed workbook for managing depression and anxiety, and co-author with Janet Singer of *Overcoming OCD: A Journey to Recovery*. Dr. Gillihan has a clinical practice in Haverford, Pennsylvania, where he specializes in CBT and mindfulness-based interventions for anxiety, depression, and related conditions. He lives outside Philadelphia with his wife and three children. Learn more about Dr. Gillihan and find more resources at his website: http://sethgillihan.com.

CPSIA information can be obtained
at www.ICGtesting.com
Printed in the USA
JSHW050948080221
11618JS00008B/63